Retirement Life
By Design

Living Well

with

Health, Wisdom & Authenticity

Printed in the United States of America

Pope, Pamela D.
   Retirement Life by Design: Living Well with Health, Wisdom and Authenticity / Pamela D. Pope
      ISBN: 1438200587
      EAN/ISBN 13: 9781438200583

All blank pages in this book are intentionally blank and *do not* constitute grounds for a refund or exchange.

To Lloyd Johnson, I couldn't have chosen better, Pops

CONTENTS

ACKNOWLEDGEMENTS

Nothing worthwhile is accomplished without the support, mentoring, and encouragement of others. This work is no exception. First, I have to thank my husband Michael for his friendship and love during this process. Nia, you are my strongest supporter, and I appreciate it and love you dearly, Sis. Aunt Minnie, thank you for having the generosity to offer a girl a bus ride. Adele Carpenter, thank you sincerely for your invaluable editorial input. Mom and Victor, words cannot adequately express my appreciation. To my spiritual shepherds Steve and Dennis, thank you for always reinforcing the importance of putting Him first. To my friends who are also authors-thanks for encouraging me to type the first word and stick to it through the final edit and publication: creating was the easy part. A special thank you to the professionals who provide support of my elder care consulting practice at Pope Institute and for offering your input with the book. A warm thanks to the many families who have allowed me to enter their lives and guide them in getting more from their elder care experiences-I am honored.

PREFACE

This book is influenced by my many years of practice in health care as a therapist and manager in various settings. These experiences are peppered by research on current trends in aging, elder care public policy, retirement, and long-term care. This book is not a novel nor is it a lengthy commiseration about the challenges you face with aging. This book reflects my hope for you to change your perception of yourself. It encourages you to realize the benefit of planning holistically and thus prompt change in the elder care system. I trust you will appreciate my broader purpose. There are parts that will spur you to question the conventional wisdom about your roles and expectations. That broadening of self-perception and ownership of your experience are the lenses through which I want you to view this book. If consumer power is the catalyst for change, here is your opportunity to harness that power.

INTRODUCTION

Yes, there is life after retirement. You spend younger years working toward it: emptying inboxes, checking "to-do" lists, and capitalizing on earnings potential. With hard work, discipline, planning, and many blessings, post-retirement life can be long and beautiful. The hope is to retire as early as possible, vacation frequently, and spend more time with family. What a life! While everyone can relate to that ideal goal, few have a holistic plan to achieve it. The missing element in most retirement portfolios is accounting for the *stuff* of life that happens after the retirement date. A good retirement involves more than simply accumulating monetary assets. It involves planning for quality of life and addressing financial and health care contingencies.

No one thinks about the contingencies until they are in the midst of a crisis and faced with losing everything. Enough already! Stop wishing for the best and get started designing a holistic retirement plan. Despite reluctance to have weighty conversations, some things about aging are predictable and likely to occur, even to you and your family.

Retirement Life by Design will shine a light on the path to holistic retirement planning that helps you address the health care and financial traps that can jeopardize your long-term quality of life. The goal of *Retirement Life by Design* is to change your family's approach toward retirement living to that of informed preparation. I will reinforce your power as a consumer, provide insider's guidance on making the health care system work for you, and put you in the director's chair. As an elder care specialist and health care professional, I will empower you with tools to age at home for the long-term and get you started with the quality of life portion of your retirement plan.

One

Change Your Mind; Change Your Life

You spent the earlier part of life responsibly planning. For career advancement, you pursued education, sought expert credentials, and endured multiple relocations. For family, you bought a bigger house, drove a minivan, and attended countless PTA meetings. For retirement, you invested in mutual funds, 401Ks, and IRAs. What is your retirement plan for quality of life and quality of care? Who originated the conventional wisdom that retirement was a matter of bidding time at the office while nurturing a financial nest egg? It had to be a financial wizard. Truly, some things money can't buy. Like health, wisdom, and an *authentic* quality of life. Yet the most prevalent topic on retirement is how much money is enough to retire "comfortably." Isn't that the frame of reference of working so hard throughout your youth? Work now, enjoy life later. Money is a necessary resource for retirement needs, however, it is not the only factor, and arguably, not the most important.

Second to interest rates, unexpected health care needs are an imminent threat to financial freedom and a comfortable retirement--an injured spouse who cannot work, a huge medical bill becomes more than a family can afford, or a frail elderly parent needs assistance. The list of unexpected events is endless.

If you don't think this is relevant for you or your family, think again. As soon as you reach retirement (age 65), the chances of needing long-term care for health needs reaches 45%, and increases with each year. Decent odds for betting on anything but your own quality of life! I'm not much of a "bettin' man," and I would guess in this arena, you aren't either. The only way to ensure a sound retirement is to plan for quality of life that reflects your essential goals and intentions. *That* is authentic retirement living.

Quality of life and freedom during retirement years is what you seek, yet you mis-prioritize, procrastinate, and avoid dealing with tough issues inherent to aging. What is the true value of that shiny red car of your midlife dreams, when you are wheelchair bound and less wealthy due to medical bills? What use is a hearing aid if you are too depressed about living in a nursing home to engage in the give and take of friendly conversation? Where is the quality in such a life? Many people have technical tools, like insurance, pensions, and retirement funds, but have no plan for quality of life. Without quality of life, the other financial tools are mere technicalities that you would not and could not fully appreciate.

Quality of life is the essence of living. I believe it is Oprah Winfrey who said, "*Quality of life is what your life is about; how you live it, the joy and fulfillment you receive in the living of it.*" Life is not well lived without an acceptable quality. Quality, to large extent, is individually defined. You know it when you see it and its absence is unmistakable. Unfortunately, too many retirees have to experience its absence to recognize that reality. Dare I say from the moment you are born, *you are getting older.* The healthy and wise decisions you make and combination of blessings you receive throughout life results in your seeing maturity. You deserve to design your golden years with the care and strategy you afforded the many years that precede retirement.

So, how do you develop a holistic plan for aging that covers more than an ER visit, your bills, and the ability to purchase a hearing aid? I thought you'd never ask.

Ten Steps To Planning Beyond Money

1. Expect More

This section could easily be titled "get real." Aging is tough. Most people would rather pursue strategies to avoid the look of aging than discuss pressing qualitative issues. I am continually amazed and saddened by the meagerness of consumer expectations. A salesperson can attract quite a following by offering little or nothing to people beyond what consumers *think* they want to hear. *A feel good no substance message spoken with a smile and a charming personality is a winning combination by today's expectations.* This fact is reinforced by advertisers' ability to turn smart and educated people into spending zombies. For example, advertisements that suggest there are *no risks* to a financial investment or an attractive and paid spokesperson who rattles off a list of disturbing drug side effects without losing his smile. *Seriously?* I prefer straight talk and real solutions. If that is your expectation for this book and for your retirement life plan, that is what you will receive.

2. Get Tough

People have a hard time facing unfamiliar situations. In particular, they struggle with challenges that test the very fabric of how they define themselves in relationships. The son who prefers to "wait until mother has an accident" to discuss driving needs to get real! While waiting is easy, it does nothing to honor your best interests. Revealing the solution to a family crisis requires a commitment to having tough conversations and accepting honest and unpopular responses.

Is anyone talking about a situation that mirrors exactly what your family is experiencing? People in your circle may not openly talk about it, but believe me it is happening. The many phone calls I receive from families requesting help with elder care crises bears witness to that fact. Your situation is not as novel as it appears. "Hard" does not adequately describe the life challenges of unexpected disability and resulting family crises. Families in crisis surround you, and I am sure that comes as no surprise. You can talk with your neighbors, look at previous decisions your family had to make, or open your church bulletin to see daily family struggles. Life itself is anything but easy. Your mission, *should you choose to accept it*, is to be ready to defend your family and your goals against the "stuff" of life.

Time is not out to get you, but neither is it a friend. Too often, you procrastinate and attempt to avoid dealing with situations that drastically deviate from your master plan. No one wants to plan for disaster, pain, and suffering. However, willfully avoiding important conversations does not make the answers any less relevant. You must realize and embrace the fact that the potential of your retirement experience is as bright and dynamic as the effort and ownership you invest. While you cannot predict a medical crisis, given the right tools, at the right time, you can manage the realities with greater control and less stress. My goal with *Retirement Life by Design* is to give you the tools you need to construct the life you want. *That* is what authentic living is about- life beyond immediate gratification, dwelling in a place that honors the essence of who you are, and designing the best life you can have, no matter the effects of age. Are you ready for that? If you are not at a place where that message resonates with you, I hope that one day you will be. I also hope that day comes before hindsight becomes the only prism through which you are able to view the importance of planning well and holistically.

3. Exercise the Power of Choice and Control

The most influence you can have over your quality of life is to maintain control in how you manage the challenges of living. Whether you are an older adult reading this book for yourself or a caregiver reading this book for a loved one, realize there is *nothing* more depressing than *not* being in control, be it control that someone seeks to take or dealing with control losses of your own making. Control and self-determination are the only real power you possess. Without willful exercise, these are at best elements of ***potential*** power.

To the people who prefer to not talk about long-term care, I say, you have a choice. Your children cannot force you to do something you do not want, no matter how practical or appropriate the suggestion may be. Still, you have a choice!

As a caregiver you have a choice to ignore your concerns about a loved one's well-being, or you can get active and talk with your loved one about planning for his/her care. Even if your loved one is not in a position to take decisive action or in a frame of mind to help you in the planning process, you have a choice. I hope you choose to be prepared and in control of your retirement life experiences. In the interest of owning your retirement life plan; seek to think about it, talk about it, and fully understand it.

4. Take Inventory

When was the last time you took inventory and performed a reality check? People get so busy with the motions of life that focus is lost. The people and "to-do" items that consume our time and resources are simply occupying space and not always fulfilling the purpose of their invitation. Why do you tolerate a doctor who does not have time to answer your questions? *He seems so busy; you'll just mention it next time.* Is your accountant available and actively working toward developing financial solutions for your family situation? *You're not as rich as the rest of his clients, so you can wait.* Are you an overworked and under appreciated caregiver? *You always dreamed of conquering the world, all by yourself.* If you can relate to any of these less than ideal situations, we need to talk, soon. What do you desire? What do you deserve? How do you plan to get it?

5. Claim Ownership

As far as retirement living is concerned, ownership or the lack of it is demonstrated through the soundness of your plan. After years in elderly health care I have seen the consequences of a family not having a long-term life plan. Talk about getting lost in the system! Once a family enters the long-term care system it can feel like a roller coaster ride of unpredictable medical events, financial hurdles, information deprivation, and communication challenges with their loved ones and the professionals involved in their care.

For many families the benefit of planning becomes clear in hindsight. Perhaps the first glimpse of health care challenges comes from a co-worker who confides his less than ideal nursing home experience. Maybe your first experience involved an older family member but you had no role in decision-making. Sometimes you may even volunteer at senior facilities and have a good idea of which ones you do not like, but do not have a solid idea of the ones you would use if needed. Moreover, while engaging in these activities you may never consider your own needs or the needs of an aging loved one because you convince yourself that it won't happen to you. The reality is, if you haven't been introduced to the long-term care system you will be.

Regardless of how you are introduced to the complexities of the long-term care system, you have most likely had a superficial glimpse of the road that could lie ahead for the health care of an aged or disabled loved one. Despite the horror stories, pearls of wisdom from friends and family who have been there, or the planning suggestions of well intentioned professionals, the majority of people do not plan for aged and disability health care. Many families, through inaction, choose to experience the struggle for themselves. No matter how bad another's story is you are thankful it is not yours. You simply cannot entertain the idea that it may well be you telling the same story in the future-if you do nothing to prevent the situation.

Too often families rely on others to ensure their best interests. Families rely on the government to oversee health care providers and thereby ensure quality of care. Families rely on a company spokes person or salesperson to "objectively" weigh the benefit of a purchase. Families rely on good genetics, positive mental attitude, and good luck to maintain quality of life. While all of these things are important, quality happens from active pursuit. The only ways to ensure quality of life and quality of care is to plan, advocate along the way, and get objective expert guidance to make the system work for you.

6. Ask and You Will Receive

The majority of people who desperately need to read this book do not realize that need. When you recommend the book to them some of them may not be ready for it. They believe they can "figure it out." Guess what? They cannot. They will certainly stumble through and maybe get some things right. Many of them will never know the difference of what could have been. The system is complicated, especially if one has never worked in its various parts. Not only that, but the myriad elements a family must consider to be well prepared is more than the lay consumer and many social service professional have even thought of. The key to getting the care you want in any setting and for any age is to ask for help. You have to seek an understanding of the options, you have to know the questions to ask, anticipate the appropriate answers, and you have to follow through by doing what it takes to get it done. Reading *Retirement Life by Design* is a great beginning. The end is to finish well.

7. Embrace the Beauty of Caregiving

At the very least, the majority of you are potential caregivers to others. The comfort and commitment level to actively manage a loved one's care varies with each caregiver. For example, you may be proactive and methodical, whereas your sister may be less objective in helping your parents manage elder care decisions. Your life experiences, profession, education, and comfort in leading will all influence your experience as a health care consumer and decision-maker for someone else.

It is common for adult children to live hundreds of miles from their aging loved ones. Long distance caregiving can be a challenge to actively managing a medical crisis and limits the ability to focus on the reality of an aging loved one's situation.   Being a "long distance caregiver" may even affect communication and relationships. This does not mention the challenge of being well versed in the resources available to a loved one in another state. The challenges that families face are individualized but are also all too common.   Most of my clients present with the same issue with an individual flair. Some caregivers are seeking advice on finding resources and guidance in weighing living options. Others are experiencing burnout and need new strategies to make the caregiving process effective and less stressful.

About fifty-two million people provide care to loved ones 20 or older.[1]   That number consists of close relationships that span interpersonal ties: parents, children, spouses, extended family, and even friends. If you are married, who but you will assume the responsibility of making decisions for your spouse? If you are an only child, or one of twelve, who will function as primary caregiver for your parent(s)? Perhaps you are managing the care for both your spouse and your parent(s).

Depending on the age, health, and stage of life of the person to whom you provide care, you may simply provide *guidance* when deciding a course of action.   Family, social, and medical circumstances may require you *unilaterally* make executive decisions on their behalf. That is essentially, what caregivers do; guide, mentor, support, balance, and sometimes function as surrogate decision makers for family, friends, or neighbors.

Much like parenting, the user manual for caregiving to an adult is not included in the packaging. Aside from functioning as a parent or guardian, no relational role is inherently focused on caregiving. Part of the parenting role comes from instinct; watching relatives parent well, parenting the way you were parented, or committing to doing things the exact opposite of your parents. Acquiring skills as parent caregivers is a matter of trial and error. Parents usually "get it right" by the time a child is exiting their teenage years or parents get it right by the time the second or third child is born.

Given the complexities that require one to give care to an adult, the pressure to *get it right* **now** often means honest mistakes have significant consequences. Hanging in the balance of every decision are matters of quality of life, financial solvency, and medical stability. The consequences for action or inaction occur regardless of having all the information needed when evaluating options. Every family must have a **trained and experienced impartial advocate** who can guide them in getting more from their elder care experience and explore life planning options, about which the average person has limited awareness-even those who've been a caregiver in the past.

8. Give Proper Perspective To Role Reversals

The role reversal in caregiving to a parent or spouse can be a difficult transition for both parties. When mother appears more confused lately, is falling more frequently, but remains fiercely independent and adamant about not getting help, how does an adult child manage that situation without completely taking over and becoming a parent to her mother? When a husband of thirty years and primary breadwinner for the family becomes ill and unable to work, how does a wife and mother manage the homestead, handle the family finances, and function as primary caregiver to him while transitioning into the role as head of household when that was never part of their family picture? Millions of families face these crises or some variation of them.

These changes in relational roles and life plans are such that no person would willingly choose it for herself or anyone she loves. Who opts for the short straw to have her parents-in-law move into the spare bedroom because of their cognitive issues? No one anticipates developing Multiple Sclerosis. Who elects to use a wheelchair for his primary mode of mobility?

Sometimes the most important jobs are those for which you are drafted. The key to surviving these life challenges is to maintain a balanced life; not allowing caregiving to consume your health, mental well being and career viability, and connecting with the resources you need *before* a crisis forces you to make decisions out of necessity rather than careful deliberation.

9. Explode the Parent-the-Parent Philosophy

Many people say dealing with aging and long-term care is emotionally overwhelming. Parents do not want to "burden" their adult children and children walk a tightrope between expressing concern and not insulting their parents by asking questions about how they are managing day-to-day tasks.

The issues that can cripple communication between adult children and their parents are book topics of their own. I will say this about the assumptions parents and children make that preclude timely outreach; in a caregiving situation, adult children ought to be a support to their parents and never a director.   If as an adult child and caregiver you find yourself attempting to control your parent's actions, realize that no matter how old your father may be, it is still his life. It was his life at 25, it was his life at 50, and it is still his life at 75. Accept your role as a support resource and your experience as a caregiver may be more collaborative and potentially less stressful.

Seeking to control decisions, how they occur, when they occur, and under what circumstance decisions are made will cause undo hardship and could ruin the opportunity to help your loved one age on his terms in a way that honors his goals. Isn't that what a caregiver is supposed to do? A caregiver is charged with providing support and not directing the course of action. You can have your way when you turn 75, unless of course, your children actively disagree with you! And *No, you probably won't die before it comes to that.*

I am not suggesting you ignore a parent's unsafe behavior. Unsafe behaviors, like driving with less than adequate vision, need to be addressed. I am suggesting that once you accept your role as a support resource and cease to define success by how many of your suggestions your mother *immediately* accepts, you may find her being more honest and transparent about the areas in which she needs help. Most likely, your alert and cognizant parent knows she is not functioning with the ease of years before; and does not need you to iterate her functional losses.   Nor will she respond well to you dictating how she should address age related changes. Therefore, though moving to a smaller home may be practical, she may not be ready, yet. Harping on your preference for her to move, does not make her any more ready, and may harden her to your suggestions.   Further, your insistence does not necessarily reinforce your concern for her quality of life (as she defines it) as much as it gives an impression that you want the situation *solved already.*

I realize these are difficult concepts to apply when the pressures for the average caregiver are so great. The caregivers I coach and the family dynamics I observe during elder care consultations, demonstrate the difficulty in *implementing* these concepts. With a bit of work with both caregiver and care recipient, my clients come to realize and even embrace the true "power" of caregiving. Caregiving is not about taking control, it is about helping someone else maintain their independence, affirm their dignity, and achieve their quality of life goals.

Independence is arguably one of the key factors in determining quality of life. Independence is the stuff adulthood is made of; It is what we all sought and longed for as teenagers under our parent's thumb. Older adults relish their independence and do not want to "fight" their children to keep it. As a caregiver you do not always have to be right, you just need to let your mother know you are *right there* with her, and willing to help her age on her terms.

By reinforcing your support and seeking first to help your parent achieve <u>her</u> quality of life goals, you are reinforcing your family team. As a team, you may come to a solution that is acceptable to both of you and that relieves your parent of the idea that she is burdening you. Sometimes by rushing a parent to act, you unintentionally feed into her number one fear: burdening her children. Most adult children want what is best for their parent. The issues come when what an adult child is convinced is the best action differs from what her parent thinks is best or is ready to address. In providing suggestions as a caregiver, the best you can do is plant the seed of an idea or alternative arrangement, water that seed with support, and let your loved one know you are standing by to help.

10. Live in the Now and Look Ahead

Genworth Financial, a leading financial securities company, reports that seventy-five percent of Americans have no plan for long-term care.[2] In other words; only twenty-five percent of people have chosen to design a plan for their golden years. The other seventy-five percent have high hopes and nothing to shore up those hopes. Is that an alarming statistic? You should be alarmed, especially if you are in the group of seventy-five percent who do not have a plan! That statistic needs to change, and frankly, there is no good reason it should not.

A sound way to evaluate the comprehensive nature of your retirement life plan is to examine where and how you want to live the remainder of life. Do you ultimately want to "age in place" at home?

Under what circumstance, if any, are you willing to live in a nursing home? After answering questions about ideals and preferences, we can develop a strategy for achieving those goals which involves comparing your wants with the reality of your situation and projecting toward the future. *This is not a simple task.* To do it well requires a learned and thoughtful analysis, an experienced understanding of the nuance inherent to the process, and the trained expertise to plan for realistic contingencies. Let's at least get you started and help you appreciate the need to finish well, even if finishing requires my providing more personalized attention aside from the book.

Two

Aging in Place

Most adults want to age in their homes instead of living in a facility. According to Genworth Financial, seventy-five percent of survey respondents, when given the choice of nursing home or assisted living care prefer to age at home.[1] Yet another seventy-five percent of people also have no plan for long-term care.[2] Talk about hoping for the best and not contingency planning! Truly, what is more important than where and how you spend the remainder of life? Who you spend it with could be an issue, but that's another story.

It would be much easier if you could just plan to remain healthy for the rest of your life and therefore be able to live in your home happy and comfortable, forever. The reality is stuff happens along the way that can jeopardize your goal of aging at home. Money gets tight, you hit a spell of illness, or your support system starts to crumble. All of these things are realistic life events that are likely to happen alone or in combination as you get older.

If you are counted among that seventy-five percent who want to age at home, let's discuss contingencies so you can also be counted among the twenty-five percent who already have a plan for long-term living.

What is Aging in Place?

Until recently, *aging in place* was most often associated with supported living communities. You may hear the pitch in commercials or read it in retirement community advertisements: "We offer an Aging in Place model." More often than not this really means, "We have a large campus on which is every level of long-term care. You can move to this campus at one level, and as your health and independence dictates you can remain on campus and move through the other more appropriate levels of care." So you can *age in place* on one campus not within one home or room. This is the equivalent of moving to a different home on the same block as your health changes. That is not *true* Aging in Place. True Aging in Place is a long-term care living concept of not having to move your home (where you live) to receive the care you need. You will rarely find true Aging in Place in a facility setting.

Barriers to Aging in Place (at home)

There are many reasons an older adult or person with a disability may consider leaving the place they call home. Regardless of the practical reasons, it is hardly ever easy, and leaving is not usually the preference. The primary reasons older adults leave their homes are related to the changes in independence that make it unsafe or impractical to stay (including Alzheimer's and disability). Alternately, some seniors simply prefer a supported living environment for socialization or personal care support reasons.

Among seniors who are cognitively able to choose their living situation, loss of mobility and other disabling conditions are the most common reason for considering nursing home or supported living communities. Let's define loss of mobility as the difficulty or inability to move one's arms, legs, or other body parts independently or of a quality sufficient to perform activities of daily living and basic self care.

While physical ability is important to aging at home, sometimes the physical home environment itself becomes a barrier to an older adult's ability to safely or functionally remain there. Narrow doorways (less than 36 inches for a standard wheelchair), upstairs sleeping areas, inaccessible bathrooms, uneven walkways, poor lighting, and limited security features in the home can make continued home living no longer an option. In some cases, a qualified general contractor can remodel a home such that is accessible for a wheelchair or for limited mobility. It is important for a family to get objective information about what needs to be remodeled before signing a contract or paying a contractor's initiation fee. In my experience as a therapist, aging-in-place consultant, and in our home remodeling company, I have been dismayed by the shoddy workmanship and unnecessary modifications done by some contractors. Before you sign a contract get objective advice from an *impartial* aging in place consultant with knowledge of your individual needs and home remodeling accessibility standards. The key is to have recommendations that work best for your long-term physical function.

Many people do not make home modifications because they believe it will be difficult to sell the home if and when they have to make a permanent move. With baby boomers aging and certainly thinking about where they plan to spend their retirement years, a home that is already accessible and barrier free may actually be a selling point. Moreover, there are many home layouts and options to consider so that accessibility features such as walk in showers, grab bars, and raised toilet seats are more streamlined and visually appealing. If these features are chosen to complement the decor of a home rather than appear as an add-on, they would hardly be noticed by the average buyer.

As an aging in place specialist and elder care specialist, I can tell you: if you want to age at home, it is worth more than a cursory look at the variety of support options that are necessary to make it a reality. The key ingredient to planning for aging at home is to have the necessary resources and tools to maintain it.

Paying for Aging in Place

The first step is to determine the financial resources your family has to secure assistance for the duration of time help will be needed. Since the typical caregiver is a married woman in her mid-forties who works outside the home,[3] one can assume that time is of the essence and families are in a juggling act as a loved one's care needs increase. The financial cost of managing senior care and disability needs is difficult for the average family. The typical caregiver earns about $35,000 per year.[4] In addition; many seniors rely heavily on Social Security for income, which means alternative sources of financial support may be necessary to meet the costs of continued home living.

Besides the financial assistance that family members might be able to contribute, long-term care insurance and a reverse mortgage can be means to pay for support costs for seniors who choose to age at home.

NOTE: A reverse mortgage and long-term care insurance are *not* appropriate for everyone. There are many things to consider when objectively evaluating the appropriateness of these items for you.

Mistakenly purchasing insurance or initiating a reverse mortgage can cost you thousands of dollars that could otherwise be used for your care.

Long-term Care Insurance for Aging in Place

I describe long-term care insurance in Chapter Five about Paying for Retirement Health Care. Long-term care insurance will pay for private-duty homecare-someone coming into your home to help with basic self care needs such as bathing, toileting, and meals.

Private duty home health care is a level of care that can support an older adult or disabled person in achieving the goal of aging at home. But it is not cheap. The average cost for a home health aide is about $19 per hour, which is $226 for 12 hours or $456 per day for around-the-clock care. Long-term care insurance will cover private duty home care for you to stay at home as well as nursing home care when you need it--if you purchased that benefit before you need it.

Again, if you have an abundance of resources and can afford the cost of long-term care, a long-term care insurance policy may not be necessary. What is an "abundance of resources"? The question to ask yourself is, "Can I afford to pay out-of-pocket for extended care in a nursing home or extended home health care?" Followed by, "For what length of time?"

Let's look at a few examples to add perspective to the cost of care. The average length of time for long-term care is about 3 years. The average annual cost for a nursing home is about $75,000. The yearly cost for an around-the clock home health aide is over $150,000 if you pay the average amount of $19 per hour for the care. The data used to calculate the average cost of a home health aide includes the overhead and profit margins of a home health agency which are imbedded in the consumer price. These figures will vary depending on the type of care, frequency of care, and cost of those services where you live.   Knowing what you know about your resources--and I hope you have a good picture of what assets you *actually* have--can you afford to pay out-of-pocket for long-term care? If you answered yes, for what length of time are you able to manage the $75,000 to $150,000 per year expense without significantly sacrificing your daily living standards?

The conventional wisdom about long-term care insurance is that those 55 and older should seriously consider long-term care insurance. By "seriously consider," I mean at least talk with a qualified insurance professional to get an idea of your policy costs based on your situation and the benefits available to you.

As you age, the probability of needing long-term care increases, and people over the age of 85 have a greater than 50% change of needing long-term care. There is slim chance that you will find long-term care services cheap when paying for the services yourself.

Your current and projected health, your income, and ability to pay for the policy premiums, and your resources to pay out-of-pocket for long-term care will be major factors in deciding if long-term care insurance is right and affordable for you. The more complex and volatile your medical and health situation (and family medical history), the greater the likelihood of needing long-term care and the more benefit a long-term care insurance policy may be for you. Depending on *when* you seek the insurance the more it may cost (see Chapter Five).

If your resources prevent you from paying out-of-pocket for in-home care, a long-term care insurance policy *may* be a priceless tool in your retirement plan to stay at home for life.

Reverse Mortgages

A second means to finance aging at home is a reverse mortgage. A reverse mortgage is a home loan that converts a portion of the value of your home into regular income on a frequency that you establish. You can receive the payments in a lump sum, monthly payments, or a combination of lump sum and monthly installments. To qualify for a reverse mortgage typically all owners must be 62 years of age or old, must live in the home as a primary residence, and must own the home outright or have such a low outstanding mortgage that the balance on the mortgage can be paid in full.

A reverse mortgage is aptly named as it is the reverse of a traditional mortgage. With a reverse mortgage the equity in your home goes down and your debt goes up. Unlike a traditional mortgage, you do not make a payment on the reverse mortgage loan until all owners of the home (age 62 and older) no longer live there.

How does a reverse mortgage support your goal of aging at home? Essentially, it provides you cash that can be used to pay for support needs for in-home care, pay for remodeling and home maintenance, or pay for long-term care insurance which can pay for in-home care.

Seniors can apply for a loan with private (proprietary) lenders and work with The US Department of Housing and Urban Development (HUD) to pursue a Home Equity Conversion Mortgage (HECM). Through the HECM program the Federal government insures the loan. This basically means, when it is time to repay the loan, if your home value is less than the amount due to the bank, the government will pay the difference. The qualifications for a HUD Home Equity Conversion Mortgage (HECM) are related to geographic location, age, primary residence, and home ownership criteria.

The HUD program requires that potential borrowers participate in HUD-approved mortgage counseling. The mortgage counselors are approved by HUD and are *usually* connected with not-for-profit companies that help seniors weigh housing options. To find a HUD-approved counselor, call AARP at (800) 569-4287. There are many changes planned for the way in which counseling is done. Some of these efforts include ensuring the counselors are reimbursed by HUD not the company who is seeking to write the mortgage.

The HECM loans restrict the type of homes that qualify for the program. A counselor can guide your family through qualification of your specific residence. Legislation projected to take effect in 2008 will remove the cap on the number of HUD loans per year and will increase the property value limits allowed on each loan. Historically, if you prefer and are eligible for a loan amount that exceeds the government limits, you may consider working with a private lender, but for greater cost.

If I had a dime for every reverse mortgage commercial that airs, I could fund my own retirement plan. You have certainly seen the commercials stating "you can never lose your home" with a reverse mortgage. *Technically*, this is correct. Be certain to understand the borrower obligations for the reverse mortgage because if you do not meet your obligations, the loan may be payable in full before you planned to move or sell the home. You can decide for yourself if experiencing foreclosure or having to sell the home before you are ready can be defined as "losing your home." Some such scenarios that may trigger a default include not living in the home as your primary residence, neglecting to pay property taxes (which puts a tax lien on the house and jeopardizes the lender's interests), or not keeping home insurance coverage. Maintaining all of these obligations assures the lender that the value of your home will be sufficient to at least repay the full loan amount that is due. Each loan contract will highlight the specific borrower obligations, terms of default, and other facts related to your specific situation.

If you default on your borrower obligations and do not have the funds (from reverse mortgage installments or personal resources) to make tax and insurance obligations current or repay the mortgage, you may be required to sell the home to repay the loan. *Consumer protections in the HECM loan provide procedural safeguards to avoid this scenario.* Impartial HUD mortgage counseling is important for consumers to clearly understand their obligations to avoid foreclosure or premature repayment of the loan.

When is a good time to consider a reverse mortgage? It depends in large part on your age and your goals. The older you are the more equity you probably have in your home and the more you are able to borrow against that equity. If you are a younger senior citizen (though over 62), and meet the home ownership criteria, a chronic or degenerative health condition *might* make a reverse mortgage more appealing to you. Please note: the specifics of your situation may make a reverse mortgage unwise for you. *Do not* make a decision to initiate a reverse mortgage based solely on sleek advertising or desperation for funds. If you are uncertain if a reverse mortgage is right for you, before you sign a contract seek impartial guidance to explore your options.

A Little Bit of This and A Little Bit of That

A concern is for brokers and agents to sell multiple products to seniors. Some brokers and agents hold certifications that allow them to legitimately sell multiple products. In some instances, these products can be complementary to a holistic financial portfolio. Buying insurance and investment advice from one source, that you trust, seems smart.

While most agents and brokers are honorable, there is the opportunity to capitalize on the consumer disadvantage against the knowledge of a seller. Let's face it, the average consumer relies heavily on product salespeople to determine if they should purchase. Sometimes if a salesperson doesn't have a consumer's best interest at heart, the buyer is none the wiser. There is documented case of misuse of consumer trust. Don't go it alone. Get objective guidance before you invest.

Before committing to purchase multiple products, families should talk with their financial advisor, attorney, and elder care specialist to evaluate the necessity of changing their retirement portfolio. If you don't already have advisors who are knowledgeable about reverse mortgages and long-term care insurance, get impartial assistance *before* you make a decision. The best case scenario is the salesman's recommendation is adequate; the worst that can happen is unpleasant enough that we won't mention it by name.

Some tips you can use and questions to ask when talking with an agent include:

1. Why is this product better than the other available products? Please, do not accept, platitudes like: "it is a great product for you," "it is one of the best products available," or "it has worked for countless other people in your situation." Great for the product. Good for them. How and most importantly *why* does it work for your situation and specific needs (cost, age, and timeframes)?

2. Is the agent or broker licensed or certified to sell the products they recommend? If so by whom? A certification offered by an employer is not an objective measure of expertise.

3. If the referral to purchase an additional product is to a business associate, what is the "finder's fee" to the agent for generating the referral?

4. What are the qualifications of the person to whom you are referred? Are they certified, licensed, and by what third party to sell the product recommended? Such credentials should come from government agencies, professional associations, or regulatory entities. Even with credentials, consumers must use their own discernment and confirmation with *independent objective advisors* before making significant financial decisions. An independent and objective advisor is one whom will not benefit in a financial or relational way by your purchasing or not purchasing the product of discussion.

5.   When, exactly, and on what schedule will you receive payments or benefits from recommended financial investment products? Age 65 is not a good time to invest in an annuity that won't pay anything for years.

The cardinal rule is: *If it doesn't feel right don't do it, yet, if at all.* Discerning the "truth" in the responses to the list of questions requires you to know more than a cursory amount about reverse mortgages and annuities. It also requires your being willing to walk away from "the nice salesman who reminds me of my grandson." That is where the input of objective personal advisors benefits you. A reverse mortgage is a resource that can make the difference between staying at home and having to move to a facility. Do not allow a few "bad actors" to preclude your considering this option for your retirement plan. The reverse mortgage can be a very positive and useful financial tool. In addition, when you are considering a reverse mortgage or any other product, report unethical behavior to protect others from injury. Your state's insurance department can field complaints and questions about an agent pressuring you to sign a contract, not answering questions, or aggressively selling multiple products that you have declined.

People Support Resources

As I explained earlier, the support that makes the difference in aging at home is a combination of money and people. The people resources can come by way of generous family, friends, and neighbors who donate their time to provide supervision, transportation to appointments, meals, bill paying, and personal care assistance. The other support option is paid support. Yet another is low-to-no cost subsidized support. I will explore these three options and scenarios starting with the most expensive to the least expensive.

Paid Support

Since the support for companionship and supervision is paid for out-of-pocket, one can purchase as much or as little as preferred. One can choose intermittent care several times per week or 24/7 care for heavier needs. If you have more medical needs than supervisory personal care support needs, a nurse caregiver may be a more appropriate choice of caregivers. The professional you hire should have the training and skills to meet your personal care and health needs.

The services each agency provides will vary. Some agencies provide nurses and home health aides on a short-term, per hour basis. Most agencies require that you request a minimum of four hours worth of care at a time. Other private duty agencies provide the hourly care plus 24 hour/around-the-clock and live-in care. The around-the-clock care can be provided on a short-term basis (for a weekend vacation) or on a long-term basis (throughout the duration of your aging in place experience).

There are other options to secure 24/7 care that can be less expensive than the $150,000 mentioned earlier. One such option is directly hiring a live-in caregiver and subsidizing his/her income with provided room and board. If you pursue this option, your family should utilize the same background check standard as a reputable agency would. You can order a background check through your state's highway patrol. For a very reasonable fee, you can get information about criminal convictions of a person you are considering hiring. The state highway patrol runs a standard background check only within the state where you file application. I highly recommend an FBI background check. Your state's highway patrol can assist you in having the potential worker fingerprinted for the FBI background check. The total amount of fees for both the state and FBI check vary depending on what your state charges for its part, but the FBI check is usually under $40. The total process can take from 6-12 weeks, so start early! In some states you can drive directly to the state capital (or where the state's Criminal Records division is headquartered) or use a courier service to make an in person request at the Criminal Records division to receive the report while you wait. A knowledgeable elder care specialist can help.

Alternatively, you can attempt to fill the need for a live-in caregiver through a trusted referral source, such as a friend or through church. Frankly, I recommend a state and national background check for any person you are considering hiring and with whom you do not have a longstanding personal relationship. Whether you prefer to hire a caregiver yourself or choose to use the services of an established home health agency, the best advice I can give you and your family is to understand the resources you have available to pay for ongoing personal care assistance. Talk with a qualified financial planner and/or long-term care insurance agent and explore the financial assets and resources you currently have.   To develop a full picture of your long-term care situation you should also evaluate the likelihood that your health and medical situation will require long-term care services. The more health and medical complications you have the more likely you will need long-term care.

Low-to-No Cost Support

Reliable options for low-cost support include your local Area Agency on Aging, senior citizen support organizations, disease specific support organizations (i.e. the Alzheimer's Association, the Multiple Sclerosis Society, the ALS Association, and many others) and charitable organizations like Catholic Charities.   The support through each organization varies by location. For a list of national resources see *Appendix B.*

Government Resources

Many regions in the U.S. have an Area Agency on Aging that is structured to provide free referral and contact information for resources in that region. Your *local* Area Agency on Aging should have contact information for local hospitals, home care agencies, utility subsidies, etc. The Area Agency on Aging also provides many no-to-low cost support options directly through the agency and its staff. The funding per each area varies as do the programs, support options, and the local coverage area where the services are offered.

In Chicago, for example, the Department of Aging offers flu vaccinations, support for grandparents who function as parents (including help with custody and guardianship issues), respite care (time-off) for family caregivers, chore workers, and personal care support. Since many of the programs through the Area Agency on Aging are low-to-no cost, I would suggest those with financial constraints utilize their local agency as a resource.

Ask the Right Questions

If you have attended one of my seminars, you know that they are heavily weighted with notes about consumer empowerment. I advise families to ask for what they want and instruct consumers on how to get it. The information you receive when you call an agency or office is as good as the resources about which the person answering the phone may be aware.

The receptionist answering the phone may not be well versed in every service or every new program available. This is no offense to receptionists, so please do not write me dirty letters. The reality is: I have gotten many wrong answers from people answering the phone at an agency who were not updated about changes on the programmatic level.

It takes great skill to be a holistic and quick problem solver. To borrow the words of one client "This [holistic planning skills] is not something one can learn." Do not assume that those who answer the phone quickly develop solutions and immediately offer solutions, solicited or not. Once you accept this quirk of human nature, you will realize the necessity of exercising your own power by asking about the service(s) you want and building an ongoing relationship with an elder care specialist who is capable of planning holistically and has a variety of professional experience that prepares her to project for current and future needs.

Programs and Tools for Aging at Home

Besides the main support options that readily come to mind, such as home health care, there are other options available that support families and caregivers in aging in place (at home), a few of them include:

Adult Day Care & Adult Day Rehab

As I clearly describe in Chapter Four, adult day rehabilitation is a type of out-patient care that is typically 3-4 hours in length and focuses on continued rehabilitation for those living at home. Some day rehabilitation centers offer transportation and others require a family to make their own transportation arrangements.

Adult day rehabilitation offers a combination of personal care, recreational care, and rehabilitation therapy for people who need more than simple supervision due to a medical situation or condition.

Adult day care is non-rehabilitative in focus and provides social, health, and recreational support and activities. The typical length of a day at adult day care is 4-8 hours during the weekday, but some centers may provide weekend and evening programs. Each program establishes its own hours of operation, programs, and activities schedule.

The activities in both adult day rehabilitation and adult day care should be age appropriate for older adults. The more progressive centers also have programs that involve intergenerational activities and animal therapy, as many older adults enjoy the presence of children and pets. If you have an exercise program, the staff at the adult day care center may supervise you while completing the program in addition to their organized group exercise time. The centers usually offer a snack and/or meal(s) during the day.

Medicare will not pay for adult day care as it is not medically necessary and is primarily supervisory and recreational in nature. Your long-term care insurance policy may pay for it if you purchase an adult day rehabilitation or adult care benefit. Medicaid may pay for adult day care. Adult day care is a good option for caregivers who work and want their loved one to have supervision and socialization when the rest of the family is not home. An adult day care program alone or coupled with other support programs, like private duty home care, can support your family in avoiding or postponing permanent nursing home placement.

The PACE Program

The Program for All Inclusive Care for the Elderly (PACE) is an innovative long-term care program that helps those 55 years of age or older who are officially certified as eligible for nursing home care to remain at home instead of going into a nursing home. The PACE program itself provides all Medicare and Medicaid covered services to those participating in the program. Most of the services are delivered in an adult day program, but the PACE services must also include home health care, nursing home level services, acute care services, and hospice. There is an application and enrollment process to participate in a PACE program.

Respite Care

Respite Care is a program that focuses on relieving stress and offering "time-off" to regular family caregivers. If you are a full-time caregiver, respite care can be a welcome relief and offers time for you to hopefully focus on your own well-being. Respite care usually occurs in the home, but retirement communities and nursing homes also offer families the opportunity to place their loved one in the center on a short-term basis. In this case, respite care is paid out-of-pocket (directly by the family) and/or Medicaid, and some private insurance companies.

Medicare will pay for respite care if your family is also receiving hospice (end-of-life) care. Yet, you do not have to receive hospice care in order to receive respite care. Respite is appropriate for all families where a loved one requires a significant amount of direct supervision from a caregiver, regardless of the medical need of the senior.

Family, Friends, and Neighbors (Informal Caregivers)

Seventy-eight percent of people who need long-term care get that care exclusively from unpaid family members, friends, and/or neighbors.[5] Most older people have a difficult time trusting strangers, especially when the person is coming into their home to provide the care. Who can blame them? Long-term care is an intimate level of care and the caregiver provides direct support for some of the most personal day-to-day activities. The emotional connection, the trust factor, and financial considerations all contribute to why most people rely on trusted confidants to provide care before seeking paid assistance.

Informal and family caregivers have an important job, and if they were reimbursed, the dollar value of the care they provide would be significant. In fact, the estimated value of unpaid informal and family caregivers amounted to over 250 billion dollars in the year 2000.[6] That is the economic *worth*, not payment, since family, friends, and neighbors are usually unpaid.

Only fourteen percent of people who rely on family and friends also use a combination of paid help.[7] This may be related to the trust, financial, and emotional factors I previously mentioned. The statistically less frequent use of outside support may also be due to a lack of knowledge about the many alternative support options I've highlighted in Appendix B. As a family caregiver, you do not have to provide all of the care by yourself.

Sometimes working with your church or worship center's senior program can help your loved one feel more comfortable and offer caregivers much needed support. An experienced consultant can help you develop a strategy to manage caregiving.

The Physical Home Environment

Let's take a look at the home environment and discuss some strategies that can make it easier for seniors and those with disabilities to get around and function within their home. While I cannot list every available solution, I'm excited to share some of this information with you!

Home safety and fall prevention are a major challenge to aging in place. Most falls happen while seniors are in their homes and while they are participating in basic activities of daily living. While risky behavior plays a role in the number of falls, such as climbing ladders or not using recommended walking aides, most falls just happen.

What room in the home poses the highest risk for a fall to occur? You guessed it, the bathroom. The bathroom can be a trap and fall hazard for seniors with poor balance and limited mobility. Many older homes do not have palatial and spacious master bathroom suites. The typical older bathroom is a tight space, which also has its benefits, unless you are using a walker which must be left at the bathroom door due to limited space inside the bathroom.

Top Five Aging-in-Place Concerns & Solutions

This list is by no means all inclusive but I will provide my top *general* concerns and easy solutions.

1). Grab bars. Grab bars come in a variety of shapes, lengths, diameters, surface textures, and functionalities. Grab bars exist that have anti-microbial surfaces, smooth surfaces or roughened surfaces for added grip. I usually recommend a rough surface, manufactured or home modified with the addition of adhesive strips with a rough texture, with a diameter small enough to completely wrap your hand around, and mounted at an angle that offers leverage to turn a slip and fall into a controlled descent.

2). Throw rugs. If you use a walker, have trouble clearing the floor with any part of your foot during walking, have poor balance, have poor vision, or have a history of falling, remove the throw rugs. They may perfectly accent the room decor, but they can trip you or slip under your weight. If you do have a throw rug at home (such as in front of the tub), make sure it has a rubber backing or underneath it place a product manufactured to stop the skidding of rugs and other items.

A word of advice, follow the manufacturer's instructions about using and cleaning the non-skid product, as the grip strength of products are not all equal and the build-up of hair and dust may impede its non-skid properties.

3). High cabinets.   Most kitchens have upper and lower cabinets. The temptation for some older adults is to continue to use the upper cabinets with the aide of a step stool, kitchen ladder, or teetering on their toes. All of these activities are a recipe for falling.

If you regularly use a walking aide (cane/walker) and have items overhead that you cannot reach with your feet grounded on the floor, I would advise you to get someone else to reach those items or seriously consider changing your cabinet arrangement.   The items overhead, if anything, should be items you use infrequently, such as the Christmas casserole dish, which your family and guests can bring down for the occasion.   Generally, the best place for items to be within a cabinet is between shoulder and waist height, the level that requires little to no bending or reaching.   If you are interested in modifying your home there are myriad high tech options available including hydraulic cabinets that elevate and lower at the push of a button.

4). Stairwells and railings.   I did an Aging in Place consultation for a widower who lived alone in his ranch style house with a basement. As we opened the door to his basement, I thought I was entering a two story pantry. There were hooks on the wall with bags, mops, brooms, and other items. On the narrow and steep stairs were several cases of soda, a mop bucket, lawn shoes, and a couple of other household items.

While everything was on one side, it happened to be in a narrow stairwell which basically meant everything was in the way!   Before I could say a word, he said "I know you are going to tell me to move this." Of further concern, there were no railings, even though the need for them was evident as he supported himself by sliding his hand along the wall the entire way up and down the stairs.

You need railings, of the appropriate diameter for grip, and they should be on both sides since we tend to prefer hand support on our dominant side. So if you are a left handed, going downstairs the railing is on your left and going upstairs it is still on you left.

5). Uneven walking surfaces. If the surface protrudes from the ground, is not level with the rest of the walking surface, is crumbling, has grass growing through it, or is cracked or rough enough that you feel it when you walk, it needs to be leveled.

There are an infinite number of other possible issues with the physical environment and both high and low tech solutions that span the range of costs. It is difficult to address every option here and the solution depends very much on your specific situation and budget.

Equipment to Make Life Easy

One of the best pieces of equipment is a walker with a seat and basket for carrying items. They are most commonly known as *Rollator* walkers and can be purchased at some retail stores. You should talk with a therapist about appropriateness before you make the purchase and also look at the manufacturer's guidelines as most walkers have a weight limitation and some seniors cannot control walkers safely. In addition to the *Rollator*, twelve basic pieces of equipment that rank high on my list of favorites are:

1. The reacher. A reacher is a device with a trigger on one end and a bipolar mouth on the other. The reacher can perform miracles! It can help put on your pants, take off your socks, put on your shoes, reach cereal boxes from the top shelf, and even bring cans of food down from cabinets. I had one client who used her reacher to change the light bulbs in her chandelier! That was a first for me, but if it works, it is good. The functionality and ways you can safely use your reacher depend on the type of reacher you get.

2. Door Knob Convertor. Many people have arthritis or other conditions that affect their ability to grasp small objects and twist. To overcome this challenge one can replace twist knobs with levers on the doors or one can purchase rubberized knob covers that covert the twist door knob into a lever.

3. Bedside Commode and Raised Toilet Seat.   If you have been admitted to a health care center or have visited someone in a hospital or nursing home, you have probably seen a bedside commode. A bedside commode looks like a metal armchair and toilet seat combined. It can be used at the bedside when the basin is inserted or it can be used over the toilet, with the basin removed, to raise the height of the bathroom toilet for easier sitting and standing while toileting.

    The ability to get to and from the toilet is a priority and is cause for angst for many people who require assistance in this area. On a funny note, many patients rejoice when the therapist arrives because they know a therapist will work with them in finding the right equipment, setup for the room, and techniques to facilitate their bathroom independence. It is a funny thing to be popular for, but patients are always happy when able to perform bathroom hygiene activities safely and effectively on their own. As an added benefit, the patient does not have to wait for someone to answer his/her call light in order to go to the toilet in a facility and can avoid having an accident at home.

4. Stair-lift. A stair lift is a motorized chair and track system that helps people go up and down stairs seated in a chair. The stair-lift allows people to live on multiple levels of their home. There are some space considerations when deciding if you should install a stair-lift. The newer units mount to the stairs instead of the wall and are sleeker and take up less space. A therapist, occupational or physical, can work with your family to determine if a stair lift is appropriate and suggest strategies to make using the lift safe and more effective.

    Installing a stair lift can make the difference in a person's quality of life. Can you image there being parts of your house that you have a desire to use but cannot? For many people who have limited mobility or otherwise are at risk of falling when negotiating stairs, an internal stair-lift can make the difference between a sense of freedom or a sense of confinement.

5. Gait belts (also known as transfer belts, therapy belts, walking belts, and lift belts). A gait belt is not a piece of adaptive equipment per

se, but it is an item I believe anyone who is bodily moving another person should have and know how to use properly. There are different types, some have handles, some are narrow, and some look like back braces.

The function of the belt is to help caregivers safely move another person while protecting him/herself and the person they are moving. The gait belt offers a caregiver something to hold onto instead of grabbing the person's clothes or arms, should a caregiver need to secure a patient during a move from the bed to chair. A gait belt is an important tool in moving less mobile people. A person may declare that they do not need the belt. But, it is every therapist's nightmare to have a patient fall. A gait belt can make the difference between moving someone securely and dealing with the consequences of an uncontrolled fall.

6. A wheelchair ramp. Do you ever wonder how someone in a wheelchair would exit his home in an emergency situation? The answer is that if he is able to move the wheelchair, the wheelchair ramp can enable him to exit safely. Some wheelchair ramps are unsafe, if not unusable, and simply defy logic. I have seen ramps that are about five feet long that are supposed to replace five vertical stairs into a front entrance. I have seen ramps without railings. I have seen ramps with wood that is so polished you could ice skate on it.

Most people attempt to save money when building a ramp by having a friend build a ramp to their home. Assuming this friend understands structural stability and construction, he is only half way there. Contractors who build entrance and exit ramps must also understand The Americans with Disabilities Act (ADA) guidelines for handicapped accessibility. The ADA guidelines are not merely suggestions. The guidelines are proven and tested access standards that should be met as closely as possible to safely and effectively make a structure usable by a person with a disability.

7. An external wheelchair lift-Unlike a wheelchair ramp a wheelchair lift is usually a straight vertical ascent and descent. A wheelchair lift is an outdoor elevator and is appropriate where a wheelchair ramp would be too long when using ADA guidelines.

The Multiple Sclerosis Society (MS Society) chapters and other disease specific support associations will help those diagnosed with MS pay for a wheelchair lift.

8. A bed or chair alarm. If you have visited a nursing home you have at one time or another heard the screech of a chair alarm. The chair alarm is an effective fall prevention device. The alarms serve two purposes; ideally, they alert the wearer (patient) that they are doing something that they should not (i.e., standing), and they alert the caregiver(s) that the person is getting out of their chair or bed.

The chair alarms are available for purchase in several varieties. Some chair alarms are pads on which a person puts his/her entire body weight, like a wheelchair cushion. When the person's weight leaves the cushion, the alarm is triggered. I do not prefer this type of alarm because it requires a person to almost, if not fully, achieve a standing position to trigger an alert. At the point someone is standing, he/she is more likely to fall.

The other and more preferred option in my opinion is the clip-on alarm. With this type of personal alarm, the device is securely clipped to a patient's clothes and the other end of a connector line is a hair pin clamp embedded within a small alarm device. Depending on the amount of tension or slack you place on the line, a person can move more or less to trigger an alarm. The clip-on alarm variation offers caregivers more opportunity to respond before a fall happens because the alarm is triggered before a person stands.

While these devices are often used in the institutional health care settings, families can purchase them for use at home in caring for someone with dementia or with decreased awareness of the risk of standing alone and falling.

One can purchase a chair alarm for about $80 and some bed alarm models are sold for about $100. A therapist or nurse can talk with you about what type and model would be best for your family, given your needs and the concerns about your loved one's fall risk and his or her ability to tamper with the function of the alarm.

9. A bidet. As a rehabilitation therapist, I am acutely aware of how important independence with self-care is to older adults and people with disabilities. One of the major concerns and causes for anxiety

among this group is the need to have a family member or friend provide assistance with toileting and toilet hygiene.

I have observed adults cry about needing help in this area and refuse assistance despite needing it. A bidet can sometimes be the solution. It is a toilet hygiene device that sets on your toilet seat and uses water to cleanse after toileting. It can be purchased with water pressure and temperature regulators and have options like warm air, hydraulic powered toilet seat, dual water spray nozzles, and seat warming. The cost of a bidet ranges from the basic models at around $300 to a deluxe model at over $1,000.

There are other water-based cleaning devices including those that attach to the sink and lie over the toilet, use a water bottle and a hose, and provide low-tech solutions like a toileting wand which basically is a long handled tong for toilet paper. If you have a loved one who is having problems with toileting hygiene, the bidet, or a version of it may be a welcome solution to address their anxiety and increase their independence.

10. The sock aid. If there is one gadget that consistently amazes people, it is the sock aid. When patients first see it, they have no idea about its intended use. The sock aid typically looks like a plastic trough with two ropes tied on the end. It is perfect for helping people put on regular socks without having to bend forward to pull on the sock using weak fingers. The sock aid comes in several variations depending on your hand strength and type of sock.

11. Elastic shoe laces. There are many reasons tying shoes can become difficult, they include increased abdominal girth, limited flexibility, and poor hand strength. The elastic shoe lace can allow people who prefer to wear athletic shoes continue to do so instead of requiring slip on shoes. The elastic shoe lace can be fixed so that a person can easily slip his/her foot into the shoe without having to tie the lace again. The elastic lace stretches to accommodate the size of a foot. It, in effect, turns a lace-up athletic shoe into a slip on shoe. The laces are commonly available at home health supply stores and may also be purchased at some local pharmacy stores. There are several variations and depending on why you need them, some variations will work better than others.

12. An inflatable bed shampoo basin. For many people, a good shower and a thorough hair shampoo are the epitome of being clean. If you have a disability and a home layout that does not afford the opportunity to get out of bed and into a shower (or stand at the sink), it becomes very difficult for a caregiver to perform the otherwise simple task of hair washing.

One of the solutions is an inflatable shampoo basin for use in a bed. The basin itself looks much like the salon basin, consisting of a reservoir for used water, a neck groove for comfortably leaning backwards over the basin, and a water bag and shower spout for clean rinsing. The more convenient models have a drainage hole at the bottom to which you can attach a hose when the shampoo is completed. There are several other options for hair washing including a shampoo tray for use when a person is seated in a wheelchair.

There are at least *ten thousand* equipment options and variations of equipment available. Some options are low tech, like those listed here, some are high tech and perform personal care and mobility tasks that are difficult to imagine, until a specialist educates you about them. Simply know that if you have a difficulty, I can assure you, there is most likely a gadget, compensatory strategy, or adaptive technique to help you maintain independence and safety. The "right" piece of equipment is the one that works best, depending on the subject matter. Determining what is right most often requires knowledge of physical rehabilitation, medical and health prognosis, and an understanding of the myriad options available.

The Coaching Session

There are additional practical solutions that may be most appropriate for your personal situation. Though this list is relatively brief, I trust it helped you appreciate the assistance that is available from a qualified elder care specialist. If you would like to "pick my brain" about what works best for your situation, give me a call. In thinking about aging in place, it is important to not only consider the idea of being at home over another living arrangement. Being successful at aging in place at home involves being able to navigate the physical environment, functioning well and safely, and being able to access and afford the people resources needed to remain in the home setting.

Aging at home is the long-term care priority for most seniors. With adequate assessment and expert guidance you can achieve your goal of aging at home for life. The qualitative distinguishing factor between the do-it-yourself approach and the benefit of expert elder care guidance is the knowledge and credentials brought to bear in evaluating options for current challenges and projecting future needs. After all, it is your life you are planning.

Three

Independent and Assisted Living

There are living environments that offer more personal care assistance and medical support than living in a single-family home, but less restriction than a nursing home setting. These supported living environments include assisted living and independent living. Independent living provides the least amount of personal care and medical support, followed by assisted living.

Within the supported living level of care, I will also include Continuing Care Retirement Communities (CCRC's) which are large campuses that offer all levels of long-term care-independent living, assisted living, and nursing home care.

Is Supported Living Right For You?

There are as many reasons to choose supported living as there are families and their preferences. Some people are adamant about not moving from their traditional homestead into a facility of any kind. However, I have consulted with baby boomers who are still several years from retirement who look forward to downsizing into a condo or active senior independent living center. Some of them joke that the downsized senior apartment will be too small for their adult children to move back home. I guess some people are plagued less by the sadness of an empty nest.

Of the older adults who decide supported living is best, the reasons often revolve around social support and a need for a sense of community. The sense of community connection can be lost in old neighborhoods because those neighborhoods change. Younger families move in and the neighboring families and friends who lived on the block "back when" have move away.

The majority of seniors' cohorts either enter retirement homes, move to be near their adult children, or a combination of other factors.

As a result many seniors find themselves among the few "original" families in a neighborhood. With so much changing within neighborhoods, seniors can feel isolated and disconnected. Social isolation is a significant challenge to the health and well being of older adults in communities that are changing such that a neighborhood may not reflect or relate to an older adult's values and needs. Supported living can offer the socialization and personal care assistance isolated seniors need.

Because seniors who are isolated tend to receive less support, their isolation may go unnoticed and as a result may escalate into untreated depression. When assessing the risk for depression in the local geriatric population, The New York City Department of Health and Mental Hygiene found that older adults in urban areas were at greater risk for social isolation and depression.[1]   Unfortunately, some professionals and the public think depression and sadness are a normal part of aging and therefore should be expected and accepted. The reality is that prolonged sadness and depression are not normal for any age and should be addressed by the appropriate professional.

While functional losses are a part of aging, the emotional impact of age related losses is an individualized experience. If an individual cannot actively participate in life's activities, make executive decisions, carry out life's responsibilities, or appears functional though chronically unhappy and withdrawn, those are signs of a mental and emotional crisis. Some people feel embarrassed about admitting they are having a hard time coping with a loss. Depression is not an uncommon illness. It can be treated and is preventable.

According to the American Foundation for Suicide Prevention:

- More Americans suffer from depression than coronary heart disease (7 million), cancer (6 million) and AIDS (200,000) combined.
- Risk factors for suicide among the elderly include a previous attempt, the presence of a mental illness, and the presence of a physical illness, social isolation, and access to means.[2]

Social isolation and the lack of a support network are a major cause of concern for the physical safety and mental well-being of older adults and people with disabilities. To address and properly identify depression, health care professionals, family members, and other caregivers who have contact with aging and disabled persons need to know the signs of depression to facilitate timely intervention.

Families and caregivers to older adults need to be knowledgeable about depression and be able to provide those they suspect have depression with living and support alternatives that may first include medical treatment, building a support network, and helping an older person reenergize their quality of life to a level that is functional and acceptable. This may also include pursuing a supported living environment.

Common Signs of Depression include:

- An overwhelming feeling of sadness

  When asked how they are doing people dealing with depression will often say they just feel "blah" or they feel "empty." It is the feeling of nothingness that indicates a loss of meaning in life. Sadness is a normal part of grieving. However, when that sadness carries on throughout the day, for weeks and months at a time, it is suggestive of depression.

- Pessimism and hopelessness

  Hope is the belief that things can be better, the conviction that they will be, and the determination that you have the power to facilitate it. Depression robs a person of that conviction.

- Self-blame and guilt

  Self-blame can be very difficult to address as a family member. No matter how you rationalize with your loved one that they made the best decision they could or that they cannot change the past, they are unable to release themselves from the punishment of thinking if only they could have done something better or differently.

- Loss of interest in previously valued activities

The activities and recreational pursuits that once occupied their life and brought satisfaction no longer have the same value or quality of life benefit. Where card games with friends or church on Sundays were never missed before, with depressions they take a back seat to frequent inactivity. Pleasures in life, including sex, may no longer have appeal.

- Loss of energy and feeling drained even with inactivity

You may find the person presents with such low energy that even basic tasks seem to require significant effort. They do not have energy to shower, energy to wash the dishes, or energy to engage in other activities that require minimal exertion.

- Changes in sleep patterns

Depression can lead to oversleeping, sleeping less, or fits of restlessness when attempting to sleep. It is almost like the person's mind is so preoccupied with their circumstances that thoughts about their situation will not allow them to truly rest. For some people they cannot settle their minds and bodies enough to achieve recuperative sleep. Others find that sleep is a refuge from their persistent thoughts of helplessness or anxiety. This can lead to oversleeping as sleep and unconsciousness is the only way they can gain relief from their overwhelming sadness.

- Inability to mentally focus

Often people with depression have a hard time concentrating on even basic tasks. At times they will have trouble following the ebbs and flow of conversations, recalling details that are commonly used or relevant to the performance of particular tasks, and they may even have problems with short-term memory, such as recalling the location of items, and remembering names, dates, and appointments.

- Changes in Appetite

Like changes in sleep, the changes in appetite can occur in two extremes. One person with depression may eat very little and show significant weight losses, due to a lack of interest and lack of enjoyment received from food. Others may find solace in food and participate in what is now commonly known as emotional eating or binge eating. A person who finds solace in food as an emotional eater may also experience weight gains. Since depression can have highs (mania) and lows, some people may exhibit weight patterns that mimic a yo-yo, with weight gains and weight losses.

- Being Irritable

I have worked with many people who were diagnosed with clinical depression and some who probably should have been but were not receptive to treatment. In many instances, it seems that no matter what you say or do, you can not satisfy the person. They appear short-tempered and generally restless and difficult to console. They can appear crowded and bothered by your mere presence and your attempts to help seem to have the exact opposite effect.

- Complaints of physical problems that do not respond to treatment

You may be familiar with hypercondriasis, the condition where people are very concerned that they have a number of conditions or illnesses. With depression the physical complaints can best be described as a physical manifestation of emotional discord. Essentially, thoughts and emotions are energy, if there is no productive outlet or release for that energy, it can translate into problems such as headaches, backaches, stomach aches, and other physical symptoms. These physical complaints may not have a corresponding traceable origin, and thus often do not respond to treatments.

- Suicidal thoughts and even suicide attempts

  Suicidal thoughts and attempts at suicide are a clear sign of mental and emotional discord. Most people who attempt suicide show signs of depression before the attempt. In fact, seventy percent of people who attempt suicide tell someone about their plans or exhibit warning signs.[3] The key for family, friends, health care professionals, and other caregivers is to recognize warning signs and make an attempt at outreach before a suicide attempt occurs.

Did you know seniors are more likely to be successful at a suicide attempt? That is because seniors employ more aggressive and forceful means when attempting suicide. While suicide is more prevalent in the younger populations, seniors are also at risk and the effect of prolonged sadness and depression in the mature adult population should not be minimized.

Suicide is not the only result of depression. Many times people who are depressed also delay seeking medical treatment for other conditions and are resistant to outside assistance which can further complicate their long-term care situation.

We all know as we age our mobility and senses change. Changes in balance, loss of vision, problems with hearing or loss of sight can make navigating a sprawling home more taxing and dangerous if not properly addressed.

Most people do not have a solid understanding of available support options and continue to struggle needlessly with challenges. An understanding of the various health and support services available to families is a way to provide timely and appropriate options to seniors, people with disabilities, and the caregivers who help in the decision making process. Some families simply give up and move to a more restrictive level of care as a way to accommodate for the challenges they face. According to the Family Caregiver Alliance, a California based public policy organization with a focus on policies related to caregivers of the chronically ill, a study of California caregivers showed that seventy-five percent of them did not know how to access support services that they otherwise would have used.[4] Seniors must consult with an impartial and experienced elder care specialist who is qualified to help them fully consider all support options.

In part, the lack of caregiver awareness about resources goes back to my original contention in this book; most families know they have an issue but do not know who can be a resource, where to find that resource, and what questions to ask to get the help they need.

A second reason older adults and those with disabilities move to a supported living setting is because of the home layout itself. Many older adults live in older homes. Many older homes were simply not built for limited mobility. Fortunately, there are simple adaptations families can make to a home that create a mobility friendly environment. We will discuss this more in Chapter One about Aging in Place.

The third reason for seeking a supported living setting is the need to downsize. Keeping a home well maintained can be a challenge for most adults. This challenge can manifest itself in terms of interior maintenance, housekeeping, and exterior general home maintenance such as yard work, cleaning gutters, painting, and the like. Many older adults live in older homes that may require more general exterior maintenance due to the age of the home itself and the amount of maintenance that has historically been provided.

Beyond the physical demand of actually completing the maintenance tasks is the cost and affordability of maintaining an older home. According to the US Administration on Aging, "For all older persons reporting income in 2005 (34.4 million people), almost twenty-seven percent reported less than $10,000. Another twenty-nine percent reported $25,000 or more. The median income reported was $15,696.[5]

Replacing a broken heating or air conditioning unit, or paying to fix a leaky roof are unwelcome events even in a wage-earning dual income home. Imagine managing this unexpected expense on a fixed income. Seniors do not reflect the charge-and-spend trend of younger generations. Still, resources can be limited as seniors live on what they have managed to earn, save, or invest during working years.

Continuing Care Retirement Community (CCRC)

A Continuing Care Retirement Community is a senior living setting that offers to potentially care for all of your post-retirement long-term care needs (excluding of course acute hospital care). A CCRC typically offers independent living, assisted living, skilled nursing and rehabilitation, and nursing home care. A CCRC can be one large complex or several facilities within a large campus.

The theory in the Continuing Care Retirement Community philosophy is that you can enter at one level of care, independent living for example, and progress through the rest of the levels of care as your medical situation dictates. Some Continuing Care Retirement Communities also offer single family homes or condominiums for rent or purchase.

There are three main types of Continuing Care Retirement Community agreements. The main types are: Type A (Extensive Care), Type B (Modified Care) and Type C (Fee-for-service). Each agreement includes the basic provision of housing, meals, use of the buildings and grounds, and its amenities (i.e. fitness center). The major determining factor between the CCRC contract types is the designation of who is responsible for the health care services and on what terms: total care, partial care included, or pay for health care as you go.

The Extensive Care agreement is a total care package for a lifetime. The consumer agrees to allow the retirement community to provide all care needs and as a result the entrance fee and the monthly rates are higher than the other agreement types as these reflect the fact that the facility is assuming all financial responsibility for that person's care. As a result of the total care coverage an "extensive" agreement is very costly. The monthly rate one pays with the extensive agreement may or may not increase as health care needs increase. So while one is in the independent living section, the monthly fee may or may not be the same as when needing skilled nursing and rehabilitation care. This is an important question to ask when considering signing a contract.

The Type B agreement may cover health care costs in part, either for a specific amount of time and possibly at a specific level of care depending on the contract. With a Type B Modified agreement, a resident's monthly amount may increase as his/her health care needs increase. If considering a Type B agreement one should take into account what health care services are included. It behooves consumers to inquire about the limitations for those health care services (limited amount of time included in a level of care), and fully understand the charges for those health care services that are not included.

The Type C (Fee-for-Service) agreement does not usually include health care services. Under this type of contract a consumer is provided access to health services but the consumer will have to pay for health care. The price for the health care services may be competitive rates; the price similar to what every other facility charges. The charge structure for health care services should be outlined in the contract.

If one is entering a Continuing Care Retirement community, there is usually a lump sum admissions amount. The admissions amount decreases from Type A through Type C. The more care the retirement community agrees to provide, the higher the entrance fee and monthly contracted amounts. If a consumer is willing to directly pay for any needed health care services, the monthly fees will be lower as may be the entrance amount. The Type C agreement is a less costly contract unless, of course, the consumer eventually needs a lot of nursing home care and has to pay the regular fee for that care. That is the risk consumers assume in signing a Type C agreement.

The entrance fee, depending on where you live and the type of community in which you seek admission, can range from several thousand to over half a million dollars. This fee is simply the entrance fee, a monthly fee of a couple of hundred to several thousand dollars may apply. In many cases, the entrance fee may not be refundable in full or in part. Your admissions contract should outline under what circumstances you may seek a partial or complete refund of your entrance fee. Remember the entrance fees are large sums of money. It may be worth it to not only visit a CCRC but to rent a room a few times for short stays. By doing this test run you can have some idea of what you are buying before making a financial investment and potential lifetime commitment of your care to a facility.

The facility representative presenting the contract should not be your sole source of objective information when weighing the total impact of entering a Continuing Care Retirement Community. If you do not understand the consequences related to signing your admissions contract and paying the entrance fee including legal obligations and repercussions on your estate, I would encourage you to have an elder law attorney review the contract with you before you sign it. Be certain to take all riders and addenda for the contract to the attorney with you. If the facility will not allow you to do that, I would question the lack of transparency.

Short of aging in a traditional home or a single-family home in a retirement community, the supported living setting that is most akin to home living is the independent living setting.

Independent Living

There are essentially two types of independent living categories in the housing community; the disability market and the senior's market.

The independent living market for disabilities refers primarily to community based services for the disabled. For disabilities independent living includes multiple "Centers for Independent Living." The centers provide life skills training, information and referral, adaptive equipment, vocational support, transportation assistance, and other support programs for disabled adults. The independent living centers can also play an administrative role in Medicaid programs for the disabled (including vouchers for home accessibility modifications to help a disabled person age at home). An example of such a center is Para quad, a well known independent living center in St. Louis Missouri.

The centers for independent living programs help people with disabilities live productively with a quality of life that is self-directed and not limited by the existence of a disability or the access challenges presented by mainstream society. The senior citizen "independent living" refers to services for seniors who would like to live independently but in an environment that is structured for senior citizens. Seniors in an independent living facility may or may not have a disability.

Seniors seek supported living for a variety of reasons, including financial, function and mobility issues, and socialization needs. For many people, supported living (independent or assisted living) is a preferred setting to living at home without a support network. Independent living is often a comfortable transition into a supported living setting. Independent living is essentially an apartment (or condo) setting that caters to older people. The apartments tend to be small-to-moderate sized units appropriate for a single person or a couple.

Depending on the facility programs, the independent living facility may offer minimal to no support for day-to-day living. Typical support services include laundry, grocery shopping, transportation support, social activities, and group meals. Some centers also include utilities in the monthly fee. Each independent living facility establishes its scope of support services and the price for those services. Where one independent living facility will offer a level of services that seamlessly transition into assisted living, others offer little support which provides a distinct line between the independent and assisted living levels of care.

Living in the Now And Looking Ahead

It is important that families understand what services are available even if they do not currently need those services. A family must also project the long-term feasibility of remaining in the independent living setting based on medical stability and level of independence. If an independent living facility offers little support, one will need to remain very independent to successfully remain there. People with unstable medical histories and a likelihood of needing greater amounts of care may not realistically remain in an independent living facility long-term.

Realistically projecting needs and the likelihood of requiring greater amounts of care is especially important if the independent living facility is not a part of a Continuing Care Retirement Community (CCRC). If the independent living facility *is* part of a Continuing Care Retirement Community (CCRC), you can remain in the independent living section, until you need rehabilitation, and then you can move to the skilled nursing and rehabilitation section, and back to independent living after rehabilitation or on to assisted living if you need more personal care support as a result of your injury or illness. All of the levels of care are available to you and you can access them as needed throughout the continuation of your retirement. Remember the Continuing Care Retirement Community agreement you signed upon admission will dictate any additional costs you may incur related to care in the nursing home and cost of care increases (inflation adjustments).

With a CCRC you may have to move from the independent living facility into a different building or move to a different part of the complex while staying on the same campus. At least with a Continuing Care Retirement Community, you may know some of the residents in a different level of care who have progressed to a higher needs section of the campus due to their own personal care requirements. In effect, you may not have to completely start over with building relationships. Continuing Care Retirement Communities vary in their layout. Some communities are within one continuous building. Others are literally spread across several acres of campus.

If the independent living facility is *not* part of a CCRC, you will have to relocate to a new facility, and start to build new relationships with staff and residents.

Staying Put

Generally speaking, to qualify for independent living a person must be able to take care of his/her own activities of daily living (e.g., dressing, bathing, and toileting) or make arrangements to meet those needs. Most independent living facilities require that a person be aware of bladder urges or is able to manage bowel and bladder needs and most other intimate aspects of his/her care.

I have worked with many seniors who require regular assistance for personal care yet want to remain in their independent living apartment. Some of them have hired personal assistants to care for those needs while attempting to stay in the independent living setting. Each independent living facility establishes its own criteria regarding the acceptability of having regular third party personal care assistance. You should know before you move to an independent living facility whether they require you to be able to care for your own needs or if you can hire assistance and still remain there.

When a person needs additional amounts of care, he/she may be encouraged to move into an assisted living facility, even if the family can hire outside assistance to meet those extra needs. Read the fine print in your admissions contract and ask about the ability to hire outside assistance if needed.

Independent Living Costs

The cost of independent living is calculated on these factors:

1. the type of residential housing unit (apartment, rented condo, or purchased single-family home)

2. the organizational structure of the management company (low-income subsidized or for-profit)

3. the additional support services purchased

4. the geographic location of the independent living apartment.

Assisted Living

In the assisted living environment you will find seniors of varying levels of independence; however, most assisted living facilities (like independent living facilities) require one to be independent with bowel and bladder control and/or management.

The amenities available at an assisted living facility will vary per facility. Typical amenities include housekeeping, group meals, in-room meals, laundry services, group transportation for shopping, individual transportation to appointments, and more.

The amount of assistance available is established by the center itself. *The devil is in the details* of the admission contract for any long-term care setting and it should be thoroughly understood before signing. I would suggest having an elder law attorney review the contract with you, to understand all short- and long-term legal and financial consequences of signing an admissions contract.

Fortunately for consumers, most states regulate assisted living facilities by establishing state health care and contract standards. Among others, the state regulations include standards regarding:

1. Licensing requirements-the minimum standards a facility must agree to and meet on a routine survey basis, including kitchen and food safety, fire safety, building codes, and resident care.

2. Admissions Contracts- the contract regulations include making the contract easy for consumers to understand and ensuring transparency in billing procedures, refund policy, cost of services, included services, cancellation procedures, and terms of occupancy.

3. Resident Care Plan-a written document that details the needs of a patient and a facility's plans to meet those assessed and

expressed needs, including activities, medications, mental health needs (as licensed), recreation and social preferences, and medical needs (as licensed).

Assisted Living Costs

Like other housing settings in the long-term care system, assisted living can vary in management structure. The centers can be for-profit, not-for-profit, part of a larger health system, or low-income subsidized. As you can imagine, the low-income subsidized centers usually have a waiting list that can be several years long.

Prior to the 1990's, unless a facility was not-for profit or low-income subsidized, many poor seniors were simply not able to afford an assisted living facility. Many states now provide a Medicaid waiver to reimburse assisted living services. The amount and types of care reimbursed vary by state. The philosophy driving Medicaid reimbursement for assisted living is that it generally costs less to pay for housing in an assisted living facility than the average cost of a nursing home within a particular state. For a senior who is cognizant and more mobile (even with equipment) but who can still qualify for a nursing home level of care, an assisted living environment may offer more freedom, choice, and less restriction than long-term care in a nursing home.

Some states require that a person be able to contribute monthly toward his/her care throughout the life of an assisted living contract. States may also require that a person need assistance with two or more self-care tasks (for example, bathing or dressing) and usually require that a person be clinically appropriate for a nursing home level of care. That essentially means that were it not for the opportunity of the assisted living waiver, the person would indeed be appropriate to reside in a nursing home. Age (at least 18 years old) and state Medicaid income and resource requirements may also apply.

Your long-term care insurance policy will pay for long-term care in an assisted living facility if your policy includes assisted living benefits.

The average annual cost of assisted living in 2007 is $32,573 ($2714 per month) for a one-bedroom unit.[7] According to Genworth Financial, the cheapest assisted living room was in North Dakota at $1,609 per month. The most expensive assisted living room was in Massachusetts at $4,753 per month.[8]

While the cost of assisted living may sound expensive, the likelihood of paying $1600 and $4800 will depend much on geography and the facility itself. The price you pay for assisted living will depend on where you live, what type of assisted living facility you choose, and how many extra support services you purchase.

While fee schedules are dynamic and subject to change, you can at least have an idea of the price for additional support services and consider future costs of care. While a loved one can enter a facility completely independent and using only the provided meals per day, needs for care can change with age and additional health related conditions thereby increasing the monthly expense.

Five Basic Questions To Ask

1). What health care services and amenities are included in the contracted monthly rate? Such as utilities and parking.

2). What specifically is not included in the contracted monthly rate?

3). How much does each extra item cost and how is it payable?

4). Is there a minimum or maximum duration of time I have to pay for the extra service? Basically, can you cancel the extra service at any time without financial penalty?

5). Under what circumstance could or will I be asked to move to a higher level of care (i.e. from independent to assisted living, from assisted living to nursing home).

This living option is expensive and complicated. I recommend a family seek assistance from a qualified elder care specialist when evaluating supported living options to ensure all current and future needs are taken into account. A thorough evaluation of this option is far more complicated than looking at cost and a desire for socialization. It involves accounting for all needs and challenges.

Four

Navigating the Health Care System

I have to tell you this section of the book, more than any other, has many technical elements that you won't necessarily find entertaining but will certainly find enlightening. I don't recommend you skip it. Just know the point here is to inform and empower you with essential information that *you must understand*. If it proves to be too much of a challenge, read it twice, or read it later, just make sure you read it *before* you need to use the information provided here.

The Health Care Factor

As highlighted earlier, unexpected health care crises are one of the greatest threats to a comfortable and ideal retirement quality of life. Long-term care is not just a retiree issue; however, those over age 65 more frequently use long-term care health services. This includes home health and nursing home care. Saying, "It'll never happen to me." is the epitome of wishful thinking.

In providing the information to help your family find quality health care, I will not discount the immense value nursing home and home health care has in the long-term care system. This is *not* about disparaging nursing homes or home health care. However, any honest long-term care provider will tell you nursing homes and home health agencies are not all the same. After many years in health care and knowing many therapists and nurses who also work in long-term care, I have been privy to the good and the bad. Like any other industry, long-term care providers run the gamut of quality and service.

These agencies provide a critical service, the demand for which will undoubtedly increase as our population ages and the percentage of Americans over the age of 65 doubles in the next 20-25 years. To meet the demand for service, the nursing home and home health industries have significant improvements to make, as do the regulators and legislators who provide the oversight.

Chances are the system won't get markedly better before you need this level of care for yourself or a loved one. Therefore, while I appreciate the value of long-term care providers, the goal is to help you connect with providers who are good stewards of the resources and health care of older generations and vulnerable populations.

This discussion *is* about achieving your long-term care goals and contingency planning for the unexpected or least desirable. A plan is not a good one unless it fully considers the worst-case scenario. A plan that does not consider contingencies is a plan in name only.

The Long-term Care Concept

Long-term care (LTC) is one of the least favored topics for the very people who most need to have the conversation, adult children and their parents. Talking about long-term care in general may be second only to nursing homes in particular, which I will cover in more detail in Chapter Six. For now, let's focus on long-term care in general. What is it about long-term care that scares people so and makes them avoid the topic? For some "It's depressing!" or many "…just don't want to think about it." If those statements resonate with you, consider what is at stake here——your health, well-being, and quality of life.

Part of the angst and avoidance related to long-term care may be a result of its muddled definition. Since long-term care is informally, and incompletely, used to describe post-hospital services to the elderly, most people make a direct correlation between long-term care and nursing homes. While the two are associated, long-term care is *not* interchangeable with the nursing home level of care. So what is long-term care? According to the US Department of Health and Human Services, Long-term care is the:

> "Range of medical and/or social services designed to help people who have disabilities or chronic care needs. Services may be short- or long-term and may be provided in a person's home, in the community, or in residential

facilities (e.g., nursing homes or assisted living facilities)."

Actually long-term care is an umbrella term under which specific levels of care and services are provided for disability and/or chronic needs. In contrast, the acute care (hospital) system functions to address new onset medical conditions or new aggravations of an existing illness or condition.

The Continuum of Care

In discussing the continuum of care (spectrum of available care options), let's categorize the levels of care by patient need. These categories include wellness, acute care, rehabilitation, home care, and end-of-life care. People enter each level of care from a variety of settings and as a result of various medical, health, and social circumstances. While people enter the long-term care system at different ages, stages in life, health levels, and care settings (hospital or home), long-term care spans several settings near the end of the continuum of care, with acute (hospital) care at the beginning. *End-of-Life* care (hospice) is obviously the very last step in the continuum of care and we will discuss hospice and end-of-life care later in this chapter. See Appendix A which highlights the continuum of care.

The Levels of Care

The levels of care are essentially, the various "places" one can receive care along the continuum of care. Wellness, for the sake of illustration, is the point at which one is not currently receiving medical or health care services for an illness or at most is participating in routine wellness checks with a primary care physician.

The next theoretical step in the continuum is acute care (hospital, physician treatment, or medical center). The hospital, physician's office, or medical center is required when one actively seeks treatment or is seen on an emergency basis to address an uncontrolled and unmanaged medical situation or crisis. Rehabilitation level of care is the point at which one receives therapeutic services to remediate, correct, or accommodate for an injury or malady.

Rehabilitation Level of Care

After an illness is controlled by medication or other treatment, one may move in the continuum to a post-acute or rehabilitation level of care. The medical or health crisis has been controlled or is currently being managed but one is well enough to tolerate therapy in anticipation of returning to a previous level of functional independence (i.e. returning to the previous level of ability or to the same living situation). The primary reason for being at the rehabilitation level of care is the need to improve strength and recover losses that resulted from the acute care experience.

During my professional therapy studies, I recall a Kinesiology instructor informing us that for every day in the hospital one loses about ten percent of overall strength. This is why the therapists visit your loved ones even in the ICU. Imagine how weak even a physically fit person would be after four days in a hospital bed. If a 40-year-old can be weakened, imagine the affect of bed rest and immobility on a 70-year-old. Hospitalization can significantly reduce a person's ability to care for him/herself in even the most basic activities of daily living (ADLs).

Rehabilitation can occur both inside the hospital and outside the hospital setting. It can occur in the hospital environment in a Transitional Care Unit (TCU), in an in-hospital Acute Rehabilitation Unit or in the community in a skilled nursing and rehabilitation unit, outpatient rehabilitation, or an adult day rehabilitation center. Let me explain.

Transitional Care Unit

A Transitional Care Unit (TCU) is basically a stop point between acute care and the next level of care. For some people a brief TCU stay, typical length of stay being 7-14 days, is enough to get them ready to return home with or without additional rehabilitation. For others, transitional care is a buffer before they move to a more intensive rehabilitation setting such as a free standing skilled nursing and rehabilitation facility (SNF) or an Acute Rehabilitation Unit.

After considerable experience in both settings I tend to favor a transitional care unit over a community skilled nursing facility, especially for those who need very brief rehabilitation stays.

I prefer a Transitional Care Unit for the following reasons:
1. Staffing patterns
2. Easy access to specialists
3. More highly trained staff

Transitional care units are most often an integrated part of the hospital environment. The transitional care units in hospitals tend to be smaller than a community skilled nursing and rehabilitation center and the staffing patterns of a hospital tend to carry over into the transitional care unit.

One of the major complaints with community skilled nursing and rehabilitation facilities is low staffing. Government regulations establish *minimum* levels of staff to patient ratios. A minimum level is not necessarily an adequate amount of staff; it is simply the least amount of staff that is acceptable from a regulatory standpoint. These staffing minimum standards vary based on the state in which one resides, the time of day, and classification of the facility as Medicare and/or Medicaid certified. Night staffing patterns (11 p.m. – 7 a.m.) are lower than day (7 a.m. – 3 p.m.) and evening (3 p.m. – 11 p.m.) staffing patterns. In theory patients are less active and therefore require less staff to tend to them during the evening hours. In a hospital and therefore Transitional Care Unit, the staffing patterns seem to reflect that of the hospital in general where patients benefit from high amounts of nurse involvement in addition to care by nurse aides.

Secondly, in a transitional care unit, patients and the nurses and therapists who work with them, have easier access to the physicians who are directing the care. If, for example, a patient complains of symptoms that suggest a blood clot in the legs, a staff person can confer with the nurses, but also can easily have the doctor observe the patient herself because she or one of her physician assistants or partners is usually in the building. It is not always necessary for a doctor to see a patient to rule out a complication. Even if a doctor would like the staff to follow-up with an ultrasound, the radiology department is within the hospital building. In the transitional care unit, a patient can get easy access to test results. When you have a volatile medical situation, quick turn around can be a good thing!

Lastly, because the hospital staff tends to deal with everything from traumas to surgeries to the flu, the staff is typically versed in a variety of illnesses. The various and complex medical diagnoses that occur within a hospital environment requires staff at all levels, including the direct care (nurse's aide) staff, to be better trained in diverse medical complications.

For example, In a Top 10 Level 1 trauma center in Chicago, the transitional care unit therapists also work in the Intensive Care Unit, on the orthopedic surgery floor, on the general surgery units, on the acute rehabilitation unit and on specialist teams including the Lymphedema team. As a patient, you reap the benefit of the staff's broad scope of training in identifying problems that may not always be recognized. The broad scope of experience helps a health care professional develop creative solutions based on their knowledge and training.

Skilled Nursing and Rehabilitation Facility (SNF)

Depending on a person's situation a community skilled nursing facility may be a more appropriate setting. Please note that according to Medicare and most insurance providers, rehabilitation and similar "skilled" nursing care is a short-term service and is *formally* not "long-term" care. Skilled care requires nurses and therapists to correct, remediate, or train a patient or caregiver about a condition or procedure. For example, does a Nurse need to provide tube feeding and continually assess a patient's condition and response to the feeding, does a Physical Therapist need to provide the leg range-of-motion exercises, or does an Occupational Therapist need to train a person on how to dress with one hand following a stroke?

In theory, a skilled nursing facility is the same level of care as a transitional care unit. A Skilled Nursing & Rehabilitation Facility (SNF) is a nursing home that provides nursing services beyond routine care and is licensed by the state to provide rehabilitation therapy services including occupational, physical, and speech therapy. A patient in a Skilled Nursing and Rehabilitation Facility may be seen by therapists 5-7 days per week, 1-2 times per day, to expedite readiness to return home. At a skilled nursing facility one can expect to receive care for more involved medical conditions with the use of more medically complex treatments and procedures than your standard nursing home.

While you can receive therapy in a standard nursing home, a skilled nursing and rehabilitation facility tends to focus on short-term rehabilitation that implies a high probability of increasing function and independence. Whereas, therapy in a standard nursing home is more likely to address needs with positioning in bed, positioning in a wheelchair, avoiding pressure wounds, loss of feeding ability, and other compensatory rather than rehabilitative strategies. When appropriate therapy in a standard nursing home will be more intensive and more frequent as the situation warrants. In fact, long-term residents of a standard nursing home may elect to return to that nursing home for therapy instead of moving temporarily to a Skilled Nursing and Rehabilitation Facility.

All skilled nursing and rehabilitation units are licensed to provide therapy including Physical Therapy (PT), Occupational Therapy (OT), or Speech and Language Therapy (ST). The intensity of therapy (amount of challenge), effectiveness (how well it works), and variety of therapy (what activities you perform) will vary greatly depending on the facility and the therapists who staff the rehabilitation department. This is true for any therapy department regardless of the setting.

Acute Rehabilitation Unit

While the skilled nursing and rehabilitation facility and a transitional care unit work to help patients get stronger, the level of care that is most well known for physical rehabilitation is the acute rehabilitation unit.

An Acute Rehabilitation Unit provides an intensive rehabilitation focused environment. The primary reason for admission into an acute rehabilitation unit is the need for an intensive rehabilitation therapy regimen. The average length of stay is 2-3 weeks, and a typical daily schedule includes 3-4 hours of intensive one-to-one therapy per day with a focus on returning patients to their previous living situation and functional independence. An example of an acute rehabilitation unit is the Rehabilitation Institute of Chicago (RIC), ranked #1 Rehabilitation Hospital by U.S. News & World Report 2007.   Securing a bed in an acute rehabilitation unit is highly competitive as the care is considered among the best, most intensive, and most technically progressive. This setting is in demand and acute rehabilitation facilities have the luxury of being selective of those accepted into their programs. One well known acute rehabilitation facility reports approximately fifty percent of referrals are not appropriate for their program and therefore are not admitted.

To gain admission into an acute rehabilitation unit one must be able to tolerate the intensive therapy regimen (3 hours of therapy per day) and demonstrate a high likelihood of achieving a significantly higher level of function as a result of participating in the program. The "level of function" includes ability to walk, ability to dress oneself, safety awareness, and other self care factors. If unable to pass the litmus test of doing well enough medically and physically to tolerate three hours of therapy and having a positive prognosis, the chances of being accepted are pretty slim. That caveat, however, does not mean you should not try.

How difficult is it to tolerate 3 hours of therapy? As a therapist, I can tell you that 3 hours of therapy is a lot of physical activity. The three hours you receive with the therapists is only part of what you receive in an acute rehabilitation unit.

The entire environment is focused on a patient achieving independence. Typically, the staff encourages you to function at your highest level of independence. For example, if you are able or working toward self propelling a wheelchair, more often than not, you will be expected to move yourself within the rehabilitation unit from your room to the dining room and to and from activities. If you are working on getting dressed, the nurse's aides will probably not come in and dress you, they will give you the opportunity to dress yourself using whatever techniques and equipment the Occupational Therapist has instructed you to use. This is not because therapists and nurses are mean, though the PT of Physical Therapy is otherwise known as Pain & Torture! While you will have three hours of one-to-one therapy, therapeutic activities are interwoven throughout your day. If your goal is to become as independent as possible, therapists want you to meet that goal. Getting there through hard work is the only way to achieve it.

Though the vast majority of patients in acute rehabilitation units come directly from some level of care at the hospital, a few are admitted from home, another community setting, or a skilled nursing and rehabilitation center. One can transition from the acute rehabilitation unit to any level of care. Assuming a medical situation is stabilized or well controlled, one can return "home" with or without additional care, or can move to a Skilled Nursing Facility if additional skilled care is needed on a "24/7" basis.

Outpatient Rehabilitation

A third rehabilitation option is Outpatient Rehabilitation. Out-patient therapy is the least restrictive setting of rehabilitation therapy. By "least restrictive" I mean your daily activities are not limited by the insurance company paying for the rehabilitation. For example, with a Skilled Nursing Facility, you have to temporarily live in the facility and are limited on overnight visits and with home health care you have to be practically unable to leave home. However, with outpatient therapy you live at home and engage in the level and amount of activity you and your doctor find appropriate. You can drive if appropriate and you can spend the night away from home if you like. Your only commitment is to attend your scheduled out-patient appointments. For out-patient therapy you only receive Occupational, Physical, or Speech Therapy and you must go to a clinic for a prescribed frequency to receive the treatment. Nursing care is not a component of out-patient rehabilitation.

Typical outpatient therapy sessions last 45-60 minutes and occur 2-3 days per week. If you need therapy on a more frequent basis perhaps a different setting is more appropriate, including Adult Day Rehabilitation or a skilled nursing facility. The number of outpatient rehabilitation visits you have per week is determined by your therapist(s) and approved by your doctor. Medicare and most private insurances will cover out-patient services as long as you are responding well and demonstrating progress with the therapy program. Your insurance company may limit the number of visits you can have with the therapist(s).

Adult Day Rehabilitation and Day Care

The fourth option for rehabilitation is Adult Day Rehabilitation. Adult day rehabilitation is delivered while a person lives in the community or home environment and is akin to out-patient therapy in that you seek the services at a clinic and then return home at the end of the therapy day. Adult day rehabilitation is best described as a combination of rehabilitation and Adult Day Care with typical program length of 4-6 hours, 5 days per week. Here, one can receive skilled therapy services and also participate in socialization activities.

Adult day rehabilitation is a tool for people who have a need for continued therapy and families in which the primary caregiver works and must be away from the home for several hours per day. The length of time an adult day rehabilitation program operates varies as does program planning, services available, admission requirements, the provision of transportation, and the handicapped accessibility of the building. These factors and the start and stop times of the program will largely determine if the program is practical for each family situation.

I recall recommending adult day rehabilitation for a patient in New York. Adult day rehabilitation was the perfect solution for this family. The wife worked and the person needed supervision and wanted to remain at home instead of spending more time in a facility. The program they chose even offered transportation.

Medical Home Health Care

In the home environment, the care options include those that come to you or those that you seek daily or at whatever frequency is appropriate. Recommendations for home based programs are dependent on the professional opinions of your doctor, nurses, and therapists. Returning a patient home, if at all possible, is the ultimate goal for therapists, doctors, and discharge planners. The community setting to which one returns can be the same as the initial setting or may differ based on the current level of ability and prognosis.

Home health care is the primary and most commonly known home-based level of care. Home health care is divided into two general categories; medical home health and private duty home health. Medical home health care is appropriate for those who need regular medical intervention under the supervision of skilled and licensed professionals. The professionals who provide home health care include nurses and nurse's assistants (nurse aides), occupational, physical and speech therapists and their respective assistants, social workers, and some physicians (i.e. podiatrists and primary care physicians who make home visits as a part of their medical practice).

Private Duty Home Health Care

The second division of home health care is the private duty component. The terms private duty and non-medical home health care are used interchangeably. Where medical home health care requires the skill of a home care worker to treat, monitor, or control a medical or health related condition, private duty is a level of care that is non-medical in nature.   Private duty/non-medical home health care is considered non-skilled long-term care because the supervision to prevent falls or help with toileting does not require specialized skill.

> **CARE TIP**: Many medical centers and some community hospitals provide medical home health care, private duty home care, and hospice care. One-stop Shopping.

A sampling of typical services available through private duty home care agencies include: personal care services, homemaking assistance, and companionship services including respite care (caregiver time off).   Specific types of assistance available within the typical service areas include everything from help with taking medications, appointment setting, bill management, bathing assistance, personal shopping, housekeeping, transportation to appointments, and light home maintenance.   Each private duty home care agency sets the scope and price of its services.

Patients who do not have insurance that covers non-medical care are billed directly for the services.   The cost of private duty care varies based on the skill level of the professional providing the care (i.e. a Nurse versus a Nurse's Aide), the amount of care you purchase (i.e. a typical 4-hour minimum), and the geographic location.   The national average cost for private duty care is $19 per hour.[1]   The amount you pay for private duty services will vary up or down from the $19 amount based on where you live.   Medicare does not pay for private duty home care.   We will discuss Medicare coverage in Chapter Five.

Many states do not regulate private duty home care; though I anticipate additional regulations will occur as the industry grows to care for a greater number of individuals.   At this time the primary regulation that governs private duty agencies are the professional license and professional conduct standards established by each state department of professional regulation.

Nurses and nurse's aides must adhere to their professional codes of conduct, but there is little regulation of the private duty industry itself. That means if your state does not regulate private duty providers there are no rules beyond employment law regarding staffing, no regulations regarding mandatory training of staff, no regulations regarding the experience or credentials necessary to open and operate a private duty agency, and no set minimum standards regarding operating procedures. Due to the insufficiency of regulation, a family must be informed about how to screen private duty agencies. We will discuss both types of home health care and screening tools with greater detail in Chapter Seven.

Hospice (End-of-Life) Care

The final step in the continuum of care is *Hospice* or *End-of-Life Care*. Hospice care is probably the most misunderstood aspect of health care in general. When most families think of hospice care they have images of someone forcing decisions on them and their loved one. Nothing could be further from the truth. Hospice care is designed to provide palliative (comfort) and bereavement (grief) support to terminally ill patients and their family when that person is projected to have 6 months or less to live. The true focus of hospice is to support a family in their time of grief and help a dying person expire with dignity, without pain, and in a manner the patient and their family sees fit.

Most families initiate hospice care within a few weeks if not days before a loved one expires. In the meantime, the family and caregivers deal with the grief and decision making on their own and without access to the support that is available when they need it most.

It is ultimately a *family decision* to pursue hospice. The professionals with a hospice agency will, however, advise you of their professional opinions but should respect your family's wishes even if your family feels hospice is not appropriate. No one should pressure your family into a hospice agreement if your family is not ready.

Families who pursue hospice have accepted the assessment that a diagnosis is terminal, a person has a significantly limited amount of time to live, and the family is willing to stop all medical intervention meant to treat the terminal diagnosis. This does not mean that related conditions that cause pain or discomfort will not be addressed.

Some families are concerned about the hospice care contract they sign upon initiating services. The contract serves a couple of purposes. First it affirms, in writing, a family's decision to allow death to occur without heroic measures to prevent it. Secondly, it sets guidelines governing how a patient should receive medical treatment in a hospital, while still on hospice care. A hospice contract does not mean that "any and all" medical treatment will be withheld. The contract does clarify the circumstances for managing a medical condition that is unrelated to the illness for which one is seeking hospice care, that unrelated condition can be treated in a hospital. If one is receiving hospice care for a cancer diagnosis and then catches the flu, your family should be able to receive treatment for the flu illness as it is unrelated to the hospice cancer diagnosis. It is important to talk with a prospective hospice agency or nursing home hospice provider before you sign a contract with them to understand their perspective on hospitalizations during hospice care.

This book will not spend a lot of time on hospice. My decision to discuss the great value of hospice is informed by my experience of watching so many families accept hospice at the last minute. They struggle through end-of–life care decisions and the grief process, and then regret that they didn't start hospice sooner when they knew a diagnosis was terminal. Just know the support of hospice care is available if, heaven forbid, your family should face a situation where it may be appropriate.

We have discussed the continuum of care from wellness to end-of-life care. The expectation is not to memorize this information, though for many of you, it may be the answer to your current challenge. Even with many years of work in the health care system, I know this is a lot of information to digest. Is it asking too much to say, "do not feel overwhelmed by this information?" You do not have to finish this process alone, I am available to make clear how these concepts apply to your personal circumstance. Since you now have a foundational knowledge of the health care continuum, let's discuss who pays for it and how.

Five

Financing Retirement Health Care

The vast majority of people reading this book have or will soon have some form of Medicare or are advocating for someone who is a Medicare or Medicaid beneficiary. In this chapter I will examine the various means and programs to pay for the health care of those with short-term disability, chronic illnesses, and elderly health needs. Later I will explain qualifications, enrollment procedures, benefits, and limitations of both programs. I will also illustrate how Medicare does not pay for "long-term care."

Medicare

The Medicare program is the primary health insurance for people 65 years of age or older and people with disabilities. Forty-three million people receive health insurance benefits from Medicare programs.

Those under the age of 65 with certain disabilities, and those with End Stage Renal Disease (ESRD) treated by dialysis or kidney transplant may also qualify for Medicare. I have worked with many permanently disabled adults under age 65 who qualify for Medicare and were not receiving benefits. If you are under the age of 65 and are permanently disabled you must meet specific procedures and timeframes to receive Medicare. Depending on your situation, the process can be simple or more complex.

> **GRANDPARENTS AS PARENTS TIP**
> Disabled children under the age of 18 may receive supplemental income payments (SSI) from the government but part of their parent's income will be counted.

Medicare is administered by the Federal government through the Centers for Medicare and Medicaid (CMS). It literally takes an act of Congress to change the Medicare program and beneficiary entitlements.

A brief quiz I ask seminar attendees is:
What types of Medicare are there?
1). A, B, C, D, and E
2). A, B & D
3). A, B, C, and D

Congratulations if you stated the correct answer of option 3, Medicare parts A, B, C, and D. There are also 12 Medicare Supplement policies (A through L) which are administered by private insurance companies.

While the letters are not important, it is important to know the benefits available to you as a Medicare beneficiary. It is even more important to know from which parts of the Medicare program you currently receive benefits. Of the four types of Medicare, you must elect to enroll in two of the programs, which are administered by entities outside of but approved by the Medicare program. These outside entities administer the Medicare part C (Medicare Advantage) and part D (prescription drug) programs. Let's explore the various types of Medicare parts A through D.

Medicare part A

Medicare part A is hospital insurance. It pays toward inpatient hospital care, inpatient care in a skilled nursing facility, medical home health care, and hospice care.

To use your Medicare part A benefits in a nursing home you must have "three consecutive midnights" in a hospital. A stay of three days is close but not close enough. You must spend at least three consecutive midnights in a hospital before your stay in a Skilled Nursing and Rehabilitation Facility (SNF) may be covered by Medicare part A. This criterion is a qualifying stay, as the three midnight stay qualifies you to activate your part A benefits. The 3-midnight rule, to some extent, ensures that the people who activate their Medicare part A benefits for a skilled nursing stay have a real medical need to use their benefits.

Once you have a qualifying stay, you are eligible for up to 100 days in a SNF (pronounced "sniff"). Medicare payment for the first twenty days is at 100 percent. Reimbursement for the remaining eighty days is at an 80/20 split between Medicare and you, respectively. If you have a secondary insurance or Medicare supplement insurance, that insurance will cover the twenty percent on your behalf. Some insurance supplements do not cover the twenty percent patient responsibility in its entirety. If the insurance partially covers the co-pay amount, a family is responsible for the difference.

Notice that when I described the 100 days in a SNF, I said "eligible" for 100 days, not "entitled to" or "guaranteed." Many families mistakenly think they definitely have three months of care in a Skilled Nursing Facility, guaranteed. The reality is you are eligible for *up to* 100 days as long as it is medically necessary and you require a skilled nursing (24/7) level of care.

Your doctor in conjunction with your nurses, occupational, physical, and speech therapists, will continually monitor your status and determine when you no longer need to remain an in-patient in a Skilled Nursing Facility. Moreover, the facility in which you choose to receive care must be certified to accept Medicare payments. A Medicare certified facility has sought license to accept Medicare and assures Medicare and the state that it can and will meet the Federal Medicare and state/local standards for a nursing facility. These standards include the facility's procedures, structure, minimum staffing requirements, and Medicare specific billing requirements, among others. Medicare certification is the only way a facility can care for patients who have Medicare health insurance.

Medicare part B

Medicare part B is a medical insurance that pays for out-patient services including physician office visits, out-patient surgical procedures, therapy when one is a permanent resident of a nursing home, outpatient rehabilitation, and certain types of durable medical equipment (DME). The equipment Medicare covers is not personal care equipment such as shower chairs, bath sponges, sock aides, or shoe horns. These personal care items are not medically necessary and are therefore not covered by Medicare.

Durable Medical Equipment (DME) is considered medically necessary. Examples of these items include: walkers, canes, wheelchairs, a bedside commode, oxygen tanks & tubing, power chairs and scooters, and diabetic supplies (glucose monitors). Further, Medicare part B will only pay for these items if you live in the community, not in a nursing home. If you live in a nursing home, the facility is responsible for supplying these items. Most facilities have manual wheelchairs already available. Given the expense of power chairs and scooters, I would not count on getting a new one if you live in a nursing home. Medicare will reimburse for a new or refitted wheelchair or walker every five years as medically necessary. The medical supply company that provides your Durable Medical Equipment can guide you through the process of refitting. A rehabilitation therapist experienced in wheelchair fitting can help you choose a wheelchair that is best for your current motor skills and projected future needs.

CARE TIP: If you consider moving to a nursing home and need a new or updated power wheelchair or scooter use that Medicare benefit before you move to the nursing home.

Medicare part C

Medicare part C is the Medicare Advantage private health insurance program. If you are Medicare eligible and have not chosen to be in a Medicare Advantage plan you are enrolled in Traditional Medicare. Medicare Advantage offers the same benefits as Traditional Medicare parts A and B. The Medicare Advantage plans can offer additional savings and benefits depending on your personal situation. However, beneficiaries may pay extra fees for the added services in addition to the Medicare Advantage premiums.

The majority of Medicare beneficiaries are enrolled in Traditional Medicare. The ratio is about eighty percent, versus about twenty percent of beneficiaries enrolled in a Medicare Advantage plan. The Medicare Advantage plan issues its own card that replaces your Traditional Medicare card as proof of insurance. Even if you are in a Medicare Advantage plan, keep your Traditional Medicare card. *Circumstances may encourage you to switch back to the traditional Medicare plan.*

Why would someone choose a Medicare Advantage plan? The plans can offer more savings depending on your personal health, geographic situation and the benefits you elect to receive. For example, traditional Medicare does not pay for routine dental care, or routine vision and hearing screenings. Your Medicare Advantage plan may cover those services. In addition, some Medicare Advantage plans have a prescription drug plan built-in.

You are no longer able to switch from a Medicare Advantage Plan on demand. "open enrollment" is the time where you are able to switch plans. The time is generally from November through the end of each calendar year. You can confirm your plan's open enrollment season by calling the customer service number on the back of your insurance card. If you are both Medicare and Medicaid eligible, you can switch plans at anytime. The available plans vary from state to state.

Medicare part D

Medicare part D is the prescription drug plan signed into law by President George W. Bush in 2003. The prescription drug plan now provides the drug benefit that is missing from the Traditional Medicare program. There are over 30 million people enrolled in a Medicare prescription drug plan.[1] Medicare-approved third party insurance companies administer the program. The Medicare-approved insurer issues a drug plan card to all who enroll in a plan.

There are many prescription drug plans with various premiums and co-pays for each drug. In 2007, in each state, beneficiaries had over 50 plans from which to choose.[2] If you take a lot of medication comparing plans can get complicated and chances in the program could inform the decision of what is best overall. The difference between plans can be substantial.

Re-evaluating your Part D plan

According to The Daily Health Report issued by The Kaiser Family Foundation, the average monthly premium for a prescription drug plan for 2008 will be $40, an increase of almost eight percent over 2007 rates.[3]

Most insurance plans know about projected premium and co-payment increases well ahead of the open enrollment season. It is advisable to reevaluate the cost-savings of your prescription drug plan annually near the open enrollment period to ensure that your best option has not changed and warrants a move to a different plan.

The cost of premiums--the monthly amount you pay just to have the plan whether you use it or not--will vary from plan to plan. The part of the US in which you live will also affect the availability and cost of prescription drug plans. In 2007, the premiums ranged from $9.50 for a basic plan to $135 for an "enhanced" plan,[4] with a national average monthly premium of $27.35.[5]

The prescription drug plan is a new government entitlement, as such; you can anticipate many changes in the way the program is delivered. One such change is caps placed on benefits paid initially by the program which are set to take effect in 2008. The goal of the caps is to limit the expense of the program to the government, encourage greater senior contribution toward prescription drug payments, and yet provide "catastrophic" prescription drug coverage.

If you have expensive medications or a lot of medication costs that add up over time, you *must* seek to understand the current caps for the program. In 2008, the first year for the caps, the initial cap is slightly over $2500 and the catastrophic cap is slightly over $4,000. Currently, the caps mean once you hit $2500 in retail cost of the drug, you must pay out-of-pocket unless you have a plan that covers the name brand or generic equivalent. Once you reach the catastrophic limit ($4,000 in 2008), the prescription drug carrier will pay 95% of the drug costs. Don't stick with what you've always had; I can assure you the plan will change. Call if you need help wading through the time-consuming process of comparing plans.

Low-income Seniors and Part D plans

Medicare beneficiaries that qualify as low-income are eligible for a subsidy (low-income subsidy [LIS]). The subsidy helps low-income drug plan users afford the plan and their medications. To receive the subsidy one must apply through Medicaid or Social Security.

Prescription drugs are a necessity for many people. For some, the drugs are the difference between life and death. Over forty-five percent of all people in the US take at least one prescription drug.[6] Managing the consumer cost of prescription drugs is an ongoing public policy debate. The government provides the low-income subsidy to help seniors afford their prescription drugs.

To apply for the low-income subsidy contact the Social Security Administration. To reach the Social Security Administration, call them toll-free from 7am-7pm EST at (800) 772-1213 Monday through Friday. Please remember all policies are subject to change so stay abreast of your benefits, application deadlines, and enrollment requirements.

Medigap Insurance (Medicare Supplements)

Medigap Insurance is a private insurance policy approved by Medicare to cover services that Traditional Medicare parts A and B do not cover. Examples include, nursing home and office visit co-pays. The Medigap policy requires you to pay a regular premium to enroll in a plan. There are currently 12 Medigap policies, which should offer the same benefits no matter from whom you purchase the policy or where you live.

The individual insurance carriers and the location where you live will determine the policy options. Each insurance carrier decides which of the twelve policies to carry (A through L) and what price to charge. The prices for the same policy can vary greatly from one insurance carrier to another.

Each Medigap plan (A through L) differs in benefits offered, the premium amount, and the out-of-pocket costs. Be certain to evaluate all options for Medigap insurance policies to ensure you are getting a competitive price and the coverage you need. Before you seek a quote from an insurance company, you should take inventory of your current and future needs, or get professional assistance, to make an informed decision.

> **CARE TIP**: The Medigap policy is not compatible with a Medicare part C Medicare Advantage plan.

Why You Should Care About Medicare Reform

Whether you enjoy public policy like I do, or not, it is a driving force in *every* aspect of your life. Retirement is certainly no exception. As Baby Boomers stress the system, the full force of public policy will become more apparent. Those who currently depend on Medicare and expect to rely on it for future health coverage should be aware of looming changes. With the Medicare program projected to become insolvent by 2019, congresspersons and senators must take measures to ensure the program can meet its obligations. These measures include addressing financial issues and challenges with quality of care. With the oldest of 77 million baby boomers entering retirement and Medicare eligibility age, of necessity, things are bound to change.

The Medicare program not only provides medical and health benefits to seniors and people with disabilities, thousands of American health care professionals depend on funding from Medicare for their livelihood. During 1997-1998, when the Medicare Reform of Prospective Payment swept through our health care system, thousands of Americans lost their regular wages and the Medicare changes forced closure of many well-known therapy and home care companies. The pending changes could again have consequences to employment and challenges with nursing home quality of care in the interest of maintaining profitability.

That is not to say Medicare Reform is not necessary. It certainly is. The old system of the government paying as much as was asked of it was a formula for financial disaster. The old system, surely contributes much to the current flux in the Medicare Trust. If your long-term care plan depends on Medicare for health and medical insurance, understanding the implications for Medicare reform and the challenges that jeopardize it should be a priority. If the Medicare program is not viable, how will your health and medical needs be met?

Medicare and Long-term Care

The Medicare program is a health/medical insurance program. As such, medical necessity is a defining factor for most if not all Medicare reimbursed services. Long-term care, by definition, is the delivery of products, goods, and support services that frequently do not meet Medicare's test of medical necessity.

Specifically, most people needing long-term care require assistance with several activities of daily living-such as dressing, bathing, grooming, and feeding-or constant supervision for safety. While these activities are essential to daily life and safety, a skilled care worker is not necessarily needed to provide those services. In other words, personal care assistance does not meet the definition of "medically necessary" care.

As we discussed in the Medicare part A section of this chapter, Medicare will partially pay for up to 100 days or a little over 3 months of care in a Skilled Nursing and Rehabilitation Facility, if you meet the qualifying criteria. Three months at maximum is not exactly long-term! The reality is that most people who need supported care, assistance with activities of daily living, and self-care require that assistance to some degree beyond the three-month period that Medicare part A reimburses a SNF. The typical length of long-term care services is three years. This alone is a prime example of how and why Medicare does not pay for "long-term" care.

What are the options if a person still needs additional treatment after 100 days in a Skilled Nursing and Rehabilitation Facility? What happens if one does not use the full 100 days due to inability to participate in the therapy program? Truly, it depends on the structures a person has in place to finance care in an alternative setting. There are a variety of settings to meet additional care needs; the question is who will pay for it? Long-term care insurance or self-insurance could be of benefit in paying for additional rehabilitation or paying for long-term custodial care.

Truly, Medicare is a health insurance and does not pay for long-term care. The options to pay for long-term care include government programs, self-insurance, privately purchase insurance plans, and public-private collaborations. Which option is best for you?

Medicaid

For people with low-incomes and certain disabilities, Medicaid may be the best, if not their only, long-term care insurance option.

Medicaid is a joint health care insurance between each state and the federal government. It is designed to meet the health insurance needs of people who are medically indigent. Medical indigence is an inability to afford the cost of medical care. The application process for Medicaid qualification involves verification of income, verification of assets, and general proof of one's low-income status. Therefore, if you make too much money or if you own things of cumulative value, you may not qualify.

State Discretion in Medicaid Eligibility

Each state establishes its income requirement (how much you make) and resource eligibility requirements (how much what you own is worth). The income requirements are loosely based on federal poverty measures and vary by the size of your family, marital status, community or facility based living arrangement, and the state in which you reside. A single person is allowed less income and slighter fewer assets than a married couple. Another determinant of income and asset requirements is not only the state in which you reside but also if you live in the community or in a nursing home.

The variations between the 50 states can be broad and changes frequently enough that I will not list each state's income and asset requirements here. In many states, the allowed assets are $2,000 or less for an individual, $3,000 or less for a couple. The idea is that a dual income family will have acquired more assets. In California, for example, Medicaid (MediCal), in some instances, allows additional income qualifiers for people who are aged and disabled. If your family is currently paying out-of-pocket for health care expenses and as a result, your income and/or assets are dwindling, you should seek to know if Medicaid is right for you.

Avoiding Spousal Impoverishment

How do you help a medically needy spouse get the care he/she needs without financially bankrupting the relatively healthy spouse?

Medicaid is an invaluable resource to a married couple, where one spouse has a need for ongoing long-term care (nursing home care) and the other does not. If an ill spouse is disabled and needs prolonged nursing home care (for at least 30 days), moderate-income couples seek a "division of assets" to ward off spousal impoverishment. A division of assets is a procedure that allows spouses to divide their marital assets to determine Medicaid eligibility. The division of assets allows one spouse to retain his/her fair share of the marital assets, while a medically needy spouse uses his or her share to qualify for Medicaid.

Since medical indigence (being poor) is a requirement for Medicaid eligibility, a Medicaid applicant must always be able to demonstrate or achieve an impoverished status. The division of assets is a means to provide financially for a community spouse and allow a needy spouse to qualify for Medicaid while contributing to the cost of their care.

Typically, upon entering a nursing home or at the point where it is clear that one spouse will need prolonged nursing home care, a couple may seek Medicaid application. The division of assets may become an option when a family and health care professional decides an extended nursing home stay is most appropriate.

I would encourage married couples, regardless of age, who experience a situation where long-term care in a nursing home is most appropriate to learn more about the requirements for the state in which you reside. Without the division of assets option, the healthy spouse could potentially lose all of the family's assets in paying out-of-pocket for a frail spouse's nursing home care.

The 2007 average daily cost of a private nursing home room is $213, which brings the monthly tab to $6,390 on a short month. A semi-private room is $189 per day.[7] A regular bill such as this could easily deplete the retirement funds, savings, and investment income of the average family or elderly couple.

How to Apply

The best way to apply for Medicaid depends very much on how much you make and how much you own. The qualification criteria, income thresholds, asset tests, and application procedures vary per state. For this reason, a division of assets is not something a spouse should pursue alone. If you have limited resources, applying to Medicaid can be a straightforward process. If you do not have retirement funds, savings, or other resources that might be used to pay out-of-pocket for long-term care, it may be unnecessary to pay an elder law attorney for Medicaid Planning.

However, if you <u>do</u> have retirement savings, stock investments, and real estate, it is advisable to work with an elder law attorney and a financial planner to go through the Medicaid planning process. These professionals will help you effectively budget and plan for paying out-of-pocket for nursing home care while adhering to the law (see page 80).

Planning will help you make decisions about the use of your resources without the pressure of needing to act with urgency. Haste can lead to unwise decisions that have lasting financial impact.

The Application Process

Upon application to Medicaid, a couple's resources are assessed and totaled (without regard to ownership). This creates a couple's "combined countable resources" which do not include the marital home and furnishings, automobiles, or burial funds. Each spouse's share is half the combined countable resources.

The state then determines a protected resource amount. The state uses a formula that provides for monthly maintenance of the community spouse and other provisions that serve to afford the community spouse a dignified and independent standard of living. The protected resource amount is subtracted from the spousal share; the remainder is what the spouse in the facility can count as her resources in determining Medicaid eligibility.

If after the mathematical calculations, a spouse's resources are less than the state's maximum amount of assets allowed, she qualifies for Medicaid. However, if the institutional Medicaid seeking spouse has more resources than is allowed, she must "spend-down" the excess in order to qualify for Medicaid.

The healthy/community spouse will keep his half of marital assets and any support payments, but the spouse seeking nursing home care will still have to become "indigent" (poor) before Medicaid will pay. The vehicle to achieve that indigence is the Medicaid "spend-down."

The Medicaid Spend-down

The spend-down is the established amount the spouse seeking Medicaid must pay toward his or her own care before Medicaid will formally assume financial responsibility for care. Given the high cost of nursing home care, the spend-down obligation should be easy to reach depending on the amount of assets available.

The Medicaid spend-down is required of all Medicaid applicants who exceed the asset level for Medicaid eligibility, regardless of why they are seeking Medicaid coverage and without regard to where they live (i.e., nursing home or community setting). The spend-down is essentially a contribution toward the cost of one's own care. If someone participates in his state long-term care insurance partnership, the spend-down may not be necessary, since part or the entire amount a family pays out-of-pocket toward long-term care insurance premiums may count as a spend-down (see pages 92-93).

> **CARE TIP:** A nursing home certified to accept Medicaid payments *could not* discharge you from the facility if you have made application to Medicaid and are still awaiting a decision.

If an official decision takes a while, once it is determined that one qualifies for Medicaid, the state will reimburse the nursing home provider retrospectively.

Nursing home type Medicaid

When someone has a stay in a nursing home and previously had Medicaid in the community, they must complete a form that coverts their community Medicaid to "nursing home type Medicaid" during their stay. The social services professional at the nursing home can help with this formality.

Transferring Assets for Medicaid

When many families think about Medicaid eligibility, they immediately suggest a transfer of assets to "expedite" Medicaid qualification. When transferring assets, one gives the assets (savings, house, etc) to someone else or sells it at "less than fair market value" before applying to Medicaid. Note that, generally speaking, transfers to a spouse are not technically considered a "transfer."

Regrettably, many families think Medicaid will allow them to give money away that could otherwise be used to pay for their own care. It makes perfect sense, if one does not have as much, the financial need is more obvious and therefore, one will qualify for Medicaid sooner. If done with the intent of qualifying for Medicaid, a transfer of assets can have the exact opposite effect.

One must make bulk transfers of assets three to five years prior to seeking Medicaid application. The transfer must occur outside of anticipating a need to apply for Medicaid. Most people do not plan that far in advance. Further, they may not trust that the transferred money will be used for their care. There is no valid reason to make a transfer unless you are already planning to give a gift to someone. There are other financial planning tools available to prepare for long-term care services.

They Know What You Did Last Summer

If you think you can outsmart the system and perform regular transfers or a direct bulk transfer of assets, keep in mind Medicaid performs a "look back." A look back is just that; Medicaid looks back over a specified amount of time to find transfers of assets. As of 2006, the look back period is thirty-six months for assets transferred to other people and five years for assets transferred to certain types of trusts. That means any transfer that occurs for the purpose of Medicaid application within the thirty-six months or five years before a Medicaid application, as the case may be, may result in a penalty.

Penalties for Asset Transfers

By imposing the Medicaid transfer penalties, the government is essentially asking why the money you earn should not be used to pay for your own care. The Medicaid program is intended to care for the poor and disabled. If you have the resources to pay for your care, you may be able to get care delivered in a setting other than a nursing home environment.

You will not be able to hide a transfer; it is not worth the risk of incurring the penalty of losing Medicaid eligibility for an amount of time in proportion to the amount of improperly transferred assets. When most families seek Medicaid application, it is because they need it now, not *two years from now.*

How the Penalty Is Calculated

The penalty for an improper transfer is a withholding of Medicaid coverage and can be calculated with the following equation; the amount of the improper transfer divided by the average monthly cost of a private nursing home room in your state. The result amounts to the length of time Medicaid will withhold payment of services. At this time, there is no limit to a penalty period. Depending on the amount of the transferred asset and the state average cost of care, the penalty amount can be one month or any number thereafter.

For example, Pat applied for Medicaid but transferred assets of $30,000 to a niece two years ago (well within the thirty-six month look back period). The average monthly cost of care in Pat's state is $5,000. The equation is $30,000/$5,000. The resultant penalty period is six months. That means upon Pat actually becoming eligible for Medicaid, she will not receive payment from Medicaid for six months as a penalty for her improper transfer.

Please note, the six-month penalty does not start from the date of Pat's Medicaid application, it starts from the date she becomes eligible for Medicaid (when Pat will need Medicaid most).

How will Pat pay for 6 months in a nursing home ($30,000)? She can hope that her niece has some of the money left and is willing to pay for the nursing home care on her behalf. Alternatively, any income Pat has, minus the personal needs allowance as determined by her state (ranging from $35 to under $100), will be used toward the nursing home costs, with any difference still being Pat's responsibility. As a third option, the niece *may* be able to return the $30,000, in part to reduce the ineligibility time, or the money may be returned in full to correct the penalty all together, depending on Pat's state of residence.

Waiving the Penalty

The government may waive a Medicaid withholding penalty if imposing the penalty will result in "undue" hardship. In Pat's case, the Medicaid program in her state <u>may</u> consider it a hardship for her to pay $30,000 out-of-pocket if she financially cannot. However, do not count on undue hardship clauses to save you from the consequences of an improper transfer.

In addition to the financial consequences of an improper asset transfer, you may want to consider the legal consequences your state *may* impose on those who *willfully* participate in helping someone else hide assets to qualify for a government program. An attorney familiar with laws in your state can inform you if such consequences apply in your state.

My advice on transferring assets to others for Medicaid application: **just don't do it!** An elder law attorney can help you implement legitimate strategies to give gifts to your family without penalty from Medicaid.

Legitimate Ways to Plan for Medicaid

The government has significantly changed the Medicaid planning process in recent years. Some circumstances allow one to transfer funds without a penalty.

One legitimate way to use your financial resources without jeopardizing Medicaid eligibility is a personal care contract. An elder law attorney can draft a personal care contract for your family. The title of the contract may differ per state but, in essence, it is a contract between a Medicaid applicant and a caregiver. The personal care contract will allow a potentially Medicaid eligible senior to reimburse a loved one for reasonable and appropriate expenses incurred for current or future services while functioning as a caregiver.

The state (Medicaid) can challenge your personal care contract. Sometimes courts decide in favor of the state, which means a court feels the contract was not valid. Sometimes families are successful in defending Medicaid challenges to a personal care contract.

The state and Medicaid may challenge your personal care contract if the state feels the contract serves to hide assets. The arguments the state may raise depend on the contract itself and the services the state alleges a person did or did not provide in meeting the contract and caregiver responsibilities.

To avoid delays in receiving the Medicaid covered care your family needs, or having to pay out-of-pocket for legal expenses to defend a challenge to your personal care contract, make sure your contract is drafted by an attorney with experience in drafting such documents and who has a sound knowledge of current estate planning regulations for your state.   In addition, make sure the caregivers involved in the contract are able and willing to meet the caregiver responsibilities and legal obligations of the contract. For example, if your son is inconsistent in his ability or willingness to provide transportation, personal care, or other support, as your personal care contract dictates, you should reconsider having him listed as the primary caregiver in your personal care contract.

A personal care contract may be appropriate for a senior who lives with an adult child and is dependent upon the child for basic needs, medical management, transportation, and the like. This is a relatively simple document for an experienced attorney to prepare.

To Trust or Not to Trust

There are certain exceptions to the types of trusts to which one can transfer funds without a penalty. These types of trusts are those that do not directly benefit the Medicaid applicant and include trusts for the care of a spouse, a dependent child, and trusts for the care of a child with a disability. For those who transfer assets to a trust that allows the grantor to receive lifetime income payments, the look back period is five years. A person's heirs, in theory, will receive the principal asset upon death of the grantor.

However, when assets are transferred within the five-year look back period, and solely for Medicaid application, you may be ineligible for Medicaid for the amount of time utilizing the following equation; the amount of the transferred asset divided by the average monthly cost of a private nursing home room in your state. Further, any income you receive from the irrevocable trust may be due to the nursing home provider to cover the cost of care. An elder law attorney can clarify the benefit of trust instruments for your situation.

Perspective on Medicaid Planning

Estate planning and tax law are exceptionally complex topics, and the laws governing what families can and cannot do change regularly. In addition, some specific requirements vary by state. A qualified elder law attorney who is licensed to practice in your state would be able to advise your family in managing your assets.

If you have multiple layers of assets that make it possible to pay out-of-pocket for nursing home care, I highly advise speaking with an elder law attorney with experience in estate planning and knowledge of Medicaid eligibility.

There are many theories on the function and purpose of Medicaid planning. From my perspective, Medicaid planning is not about hiding assets or maximizing loopholes in the law. Estate planning, for those who are potentially Medicaid eligible, is a tool to help your family manage the estate, taxation, financial aspects, and consequences for the community spouse and heirs. I would suggest exercising the provisions of Medicaid eligibility law as your conscience dictates.

As consequence of an improper transfer, you may find yourself paying out-of-pocket for care when you can least afford it. Without proper planning, you may establish an estate-planning tool that is not in your best interests. Further, your family may find that most of your assets are wasted in probate court fees and estate taxes instead of being inherited by your heirs.

Who Gets To Keep The House?

Though a community spouse can stay in the marital house while a frail spouse lives in a nursing home, what happens to the home when the community spouse dies or a single person needing Medicaid coverage dies? In the case where the community spouse dies, a federal mandate requires all states to attempt to recoup the cost of Medicaid reimbursed care provided to those in a nursing home. Therefore, if a dependent or disabled child *no longer lives in the home*, the state may place a lien on the home in an attempt to recover the total cost of nursing home care paid on a Medicaid recipient's behalf.

Your state may or may not actively pursue recoveries. Some states that pursue recovery may be more aggressive in the recovery effort, other states may not pursue recovery at all, and still others may pursue recovery but allow for exceptions related to hardship for the heir residing in the home.

If you or your Medicaid eligible loved one own a home, it is very important to understand the recovery process for your state. If Medicaid has paid for a person's nursing home stay, a spouse or a child living in the home may delay or prevent Medicaid recovery.

An elder law attorney versed in the laws of your state is most qualified to guide your family in understanding what may be required of you concerning a loved one's home.

GRANDPARENTS AS PARENTS TIP

As stated early in this chapter, states determine income and resource (asset) requirements for Medicaid eligibility. Your grandchild may be eligible for Medicaid coverage if he is a U.S. citizen or a lawfully admitted immigrant. If your grandchild lives with you, he may be eligible for Medicaid even if you are not.

Non-Government Programs

Can You Afford to Pay Out-of-Pocket?

The out-of-pocket cost for a private one person room in a nursing home in 2007 was $213 per day, which does not include the therapy, nursing, supplies, and medications; all the "stuff" that makes a nursing home stay "skilled." Semi-private rooms are less expensive. Still, with therapy visits at more than $100 dollars per hour, per therapy type (OT/PT/ST), the out-of-pocket cost of long-term care in a nursing home is extraordinary and generally prohibitive for the average family.

When you calculate $213 per day for 60 days of care and add any additional nursing and therapy costs, it is easy to see how out-of-pocket payments for nursing home care will leave most families financially crushed and Medicaid eligible within a short amount of time.

Self-Insuring

What asset value is enough to pay out-of-pocket for care? Essentially, you need enough money to pay without compromising your daily living standards and neglecting your other care needs. If you have hundreds of tens of thousands to millions saved, or invested, or if you own other high value assets that you can easily convert to cash, you may be able to self-insure by paying out-of-pocket for long-term care costs.

If you need care at home, the cost is about $150,000 per year for an around-the-clock aide. Nursing home care is about $75,000 per year, and rising. Given your financial resources, how long can you pay out-of-pocket for long-term care?

What Is Long-term Care Insurance?

The cost of long-term care makes the option of long-term care insurance worth more than a second glance especially for families in the middle class. Long-term care insurance is a policy for the care you need for ongoing post-hospital care. Many long-term care insurance policies have a typical waiting period of 30-60 days before you can use your benefits. Remember, Medicare will only pay for *up to* 100 days in a SNF, if you qualify. A long-term care insurance policy can extend your skilled nursing and rehabilitation stay by providing payment beyond the 100 Medicare days.

Long-term care insurance is separate from the Medicare program and you purchase the benefit amount that you want to receive in the future. The point of long-term care insurance is to pay for future care needs, whether the care is needed 2 years, 10 years, or 20 years from the date of purchase.

There is typically a lifetime maximum payout amount for each policy. The insurance company will not pay more for your care than the lifetime payout amount you purchased. Therefore, wisely predicting the needed benefit amount requires careful preparation with a long-term care insurance agent who understands the available products and policy options. You can purchase a lifetime insurance policy.

How Much Is Long-term Care Insurance?

Factors that affect the price and benefit of a long-term care policy include:

- Your age at the time of purchase--the younger you are the cheaper it is and the fewer health issues you may have for favorable underwriting.

- Medical underwriting--the healthier you are the cheaper it is. Some plans will not issue a policy due to certain pre-existing medical conditions or because of the medical condition; the premium is prohibitively expensive due to the likelihood that sicker people are more likely to use the insurance.

- The amount of daily/monthly benefit you want to receive in the future when you use the policy and for what duration of time (i.e., a benefit payout of $200 per day for three years).

- The benefits you purchase (i.e., coverage for assisted living, nursing homes, home health, or a combination of these services)

- Where you live--The cost of a private nursing home room differs per state and in Alaska is well over $500 per day.[8] Geographic cost indicators should influence the benefit amount you choose.

Planning for the Future Cost of Care

In 2007, the average cost of a private room in a nursing home was about $213 per day and a benefit payout of $200 per day may work well, depending on the actual cost of care in your area. However, two hundred dollars in today's money will be worth fewer dollars 15 years from now because the cost of care will increase. Inflation happens!

How do you adjust for a rise in the cost of care that makes a daily nursing home stay cost $400 per day 15 years from now? The answer: inflation protection. Inflation protection does not *guarantee* 100 percent coverage of the future cost of care. You can purchase inflation protection that adjusts the benefit amount to reflect the account for the future cost of care. The adjustments are available in several forms, the more basic of which are five percent automatic compound inflation adjustments and five percent simple inflation adjustments.

You can purchase this inflation protection as a "rider" to your insurance policy so that your benefit amount increases by the percentage you select when you purchase the policy. A "rider" is an upgrade that attaches to and goes along with your insurance policy.

Compound inflation riders offer greater mathematical assurance of the future value of your insurance investment. This in effect ensures your previously purchased benefits will actually cover more of the future cost of care. If the interest is compounded annually versus at the time you need the care (simple inflation), you will have more money to put toward care in the future. Without practical inflation protection, your plan will cover less of the cost of care in 15 years. Given historical trends, the cost of care is unlikely to decrease or remain the same.

The Benefit of Long-term Care Insurance

Look at this sample of the cost of care and benefit received from a basic long-term care insurance policy.

Sue is 71 years of age and has spent her Medicare benefits while recovering from an elective hip replacement. Sue still needs an additional 3 months of care, which will cost $13,500. Due to her rising issues with joint discomfort, Sue purchased a comprehensive long-term care policy at age 65. Sue has paid a little over $14,000 to date in premiums for a $100 per day benefit.

Sample Long-term Care Scenario *Without* Insurance

Cost of Care	Duration of Care	Amount Due	Who pays
$150 per day	90 days	$13,500 ($150 x 90 dys)	Sue $13,500

Sample Long-term Care Scenario *With* Insurance

Cost of Care	Duration of Care	Amount Due	Who pays
$150 per day	90 days	$13,500 ($150 x 90 dys)	Insurance $9,000 Sue $4,500*

* based on $100 per day nursing home benefit amount

As you can see from the chart, without long-term care insurance, Sue will have to pay the $13,500 bill herself. With the long-term care insurance, her policy will pay toward the $13,500 per the details of her policy. Even if the insurance company does not pay for the entire bill, I'm sure Sue would rather pay part of $13,500 than all of it. Please note, *each insurance policy will vary in the percentage of a bill it covers. The benefit types and amounts you elect influences this process.*

Depending on the lifetime payout amount Sue bought, she may still have adequate private insurance coverage available to her, in addition to Medicare, for future care needs.

Is Long-term Care Insurance Right For You?

It is high risk to think one will not need long-term care and from that assumption decide not to purchase long-term care insurance. A healthy 50 year old man may have a tough time perceiving the need for insurance that he may not need until age 70, if at all. Keep in mind, long-term care or extended rehabilitation is not just for "older" people. It is suggested that over 3 million adults *under age 65* have a need for long-term care.[9]

If you have standard health insurance through an employer, is it possible the insurer will require rehabilitation in a nursing home instead of an acute rehabilitation center? Perhaps your in-patient rehabilitation benefits are limited. Who will pay for the care you need at home? If you do not have long-term care insurance or another insurance to pay for ongoing care needs, you may have to pay out-of-pocket for that care. Do the math; How long can you afford to?

You can purchase separate employer sponsored long-term care insurance, but is it portable (does it leave with you if you quit the job), does it cover your spouse, and how does it compare with a privately purchased (and portable) plan in terms of cost and coverage? Legislators are making provisions to allow employers to make long-term care insurance a more affordable benefit. Perhaps some coverage, even if contingent upon employment, is better than no coverage.

With the projected insolvency of Medicare, problems with Social Security, and myriad pending government financing issues, a thoughtfully purchased long-term care insurance policy is a more secure option. Traditional government programs (Medicare and Medicaid) provide long-term care coverage on a limited basis and on the government's terms. If you prefer to choose where you live and have greater control over the duration of care, self-insurance or long-term care insurance is the best option.

However, if you have limited financial resources, private long-term care insurance may not be the best option for you; as it usually requires a continual payment of premiums. Low-income seniors may find privately purchased long-term care insurance unaffordable and unnecessary. In addition, people with disabilities or existing health problems may not receive positive medical underwriting to receive a private long-term care insurance policy (see the section on government resources in this chapter).

Enough is Enough

The amount of long-term care insurance one *needs* is difficult to predict. Since the insurance is a projection for the future, that number is elusive. The amount of long-term care insurance you purchase and the duration of the policy is in large part a measure of your risk tolerance. If you are willing to risk not being able to afford the care you may need in the future, you may purchase less coverage or forgo coverage. If you want greater control over where you live the remainder of life; you may purchase a practical and comprehensive long-term care insurance policy that covers multiple settings (nursing home, assisted living, and home health care) for at least the statistical average duration of care (about 3 years). For practical purposes, the amount of long-term care insurance coverage one needs is dependent upon several factors.

Those factors include:
1. The likelihood of needing long-term care (health status and family medical history). One should also consider the possibility of accidents, undetected, or not yet developed medical conditions-the very circumstances that may make one ineligible if you wait too long.

2. The amount of care one will need in the future (intermittent or around the clock).

3. Where you plan to receive the future care (nursing home versus in home care).

4. The cost of care where you live-geography affects the cost for nursing home and home health care.

How confident are you that your health will remain the same? Will you experience a freak accident that may incapacitate or disable you for any length of time? Evaluate if *not* having long-term care insurance is an acceptable risk for your family and financial resources. Seriously consider protecting your financial assets, retirement savings, and the legacy for your family by investigating a long-term care insurance policy.

Keeping Good Company

It is important to purchase insurance through a company with a long record of successfully providing long-term care insurance products without a pattern of premium increases. The reputation of the insurance company is important because companies may offer a low premium and then adjust the rate making it too expensive to continue the payments. The larger and more highly regarded long-term care insurance companies do not overly exercise the ability to request premium increases. This is, in part, why a reputable and experienced insurance company is so important. The other part is long-range viability of the company; you want the company to be around when you need to use the policy.

The assumptions an insurance company makes when developing the policy product and establishing variables to determine a policy price will have great impact on your premiums. If the insurance company's assumptions are faulty or for another reason something significantly changes within your *rate class*, the insurance company can request a premium increase. Your state insurance commission or state insurance department reviews the request for a premium increase. The insurance department may approve or deny the request for a premium increase.

Know Your Class

You could ask an insurance agent about the history of premium increases, but you may not get a simple "yes" or "no" answer. Long-term care insurance companies cannot raise one person's rates based on their use of the policy or medical condition. However, a company can raise the premium rates on all people in a particular "rate class."

A "rate class" is, in essence, a cohort group to which each insured person belongs. Your age, health at the time of policy underwriting, and where you live determine your rate class. Therefore, two fifty-year-old women living in the same city can have different rate classes and experiences with premium hikes.

You should inquire about the history of premium increases *within your assigned rate class*. A premium increase of ten percent can be a budget breaker for people on fixed incomes who may already struggle to meet monthly premium payments.

Do Not Start What You Cannot Finish

Families should also critically evaluate their financial standing and available resources to be certain long-term care insurance would be beneficial and affordable. If you discontinue paying the monthly insurance premiums, you lose the money already invested in the policy. Families should invest wisely by purchasing a policy with a reputable company to avoid starting out with an attractive "bargain" policy that because of premium hikes leaves them without long-term care coverage **and** fewer financial resources.

If the current cost of premium payments are a stretch for your income and resources, consider participating in your state's long-term care insurance partnership program or spending-down assets to qualify for Medicaid if and when it is appropriate.

State Partnership Insurance Policies

The original states participating in the partnership program were Indiana, Connecticut, California, and New York. These states have partnerships between their Medicaid program and private insurance companies. The partnership programs in these four states provide long-term care insurance policies with greater flexibility and asset protection upon being eligible for Medicaid.

Recent changes in government regulations have opened the partnership program to other states. As a result, many other states have some version of a partnership program. These partnership programs allow states to exclude long-term care insurance benefits during Medicaid application. In effect, the benefit payments received from the long-term care insurance plan *do not* count as assets. This exclusion is a good thing for families!

To find out more about your state's long-term care insurance partnership program contact your State Office of the Insurance Commissioner or the State Insurance Department. To locate the insurance department that handles insurance for your state, visit The National Academy of Insurance Commissioners website at www.naic.org and click on your state of residence to be directed to your state's insurance department homepage. When you speak with your state's insurance department, a representative can tell you if a long-term care insurance partnership program exists in your state. The question to keep in mind is "Which option is *best* for me and my family?" If you cannot answer that question with confidence, get help before you make a decision!

The Coaching Session

Medicare is the number one health insurance provider for people over the age of sixty-five. As a health and medical insurance, Medicare *does not* pay for long-term care. Remember, long-term care is distinguished from care that is skilled and medically necessary. Consider long-term care insurance to cover the cost of non-medical care and some medical care that extends beyond the 100 days of Medicare nursing home coverage. Long-term care insurance can be an invaluable tool in financing care for older adults and people with disabilities.

At Pope Institute, I get a lot of questions about how to pay for long-term care. Families who call are seeking objective and impartial guidance on weighing the options and considering alternatives. Since the Pope Institute mission is impartial elder care advocacy (not selling products) families know that their best interests are our top priority.

Depending on your financial, medical, and family situation either or an appropriate combination of these financial options may be right for you. It is in your long-term financial interests and quality of life to fully understand the better option for your current **and** projected situation. Don't make a hasty decision without fully understanding the personal consequences and benefits to you and your family.

In the next chapter I will explore nursing homes and how you can ensure quality of care for yourself and your loved ones by front loading your efforts instead of participating in nursing home selection by crisis management.

Six

Rehabilitation & Nursing Home Care

Let me ask you a question. Would you define a well spent lunch break as one that involves looking through a nursing home? Was that a scoff and an emphatic "NO!"? Yeah, I understand. You are not alone. I would suspect most people do not visit nursing homes before they need them.

Most nursing home visits probably happen as a result of a conversation like this: "Mrs. Johnson, your mother is doing well with her treatment and therapy for the hip fracture. The doctor would like to discharge her to the nursing home for continued rehabilitation in the next day or two. Here is a list of five facilities within your zip code that have an open bed. Please take a look at them and let us know which one you prefer. We will start making arrangements to complete a transfer within the next 24-48 hours."

Mrs. Johnson is thinking to herself, "*It's already 4 pm and I have to do what within 24-48 hours?*" Meanwhile, the health care process rolls on and over Mrs. Johnson. Have you or someone you know been in this situation? I hope you are fortunate enough to have never placed a loved one in a nursing home for a short- or long-term stay. I also hope you never have to without already knowing which facility you feel confident choosing. The pressure at such a time is immense because of the magnitude of the decision and the time crunch under which you are placed.

Discharge planners at hospitals, trauma centers in particular, have a fast paced and often thankless job. On one hand they have to help patients transition from the hospital into the next level of care. On the other hand they have new patients rushing to fill a bed within an hour of a patient leaving. That does not provide much consolation to families who are commanded to find a nursing home in 24-48 hours. It will hopefully soften the impact to your family's sensibilities to know that the discharge planners are not out to make your life harder.

Older adults frequently talk about hospital stays for events that now are same-day surgeries. Childbirth used to require several weeks in the hospital. Now even mothers with physical complications for themselves after childbirth are discharged within a few days. Depending on the circumstances, their infant may remain in the hospital, but a mother may be discharged. With advances in the way surgeries are performed, increased training and specialization of hospital staff, the prevalence of HMO's and other managed care agencies, and a much broader health care continuum, hospital stays are not what they used to be. Short lengths of hospital stays and short discharge notices are simply the nature of the beast.

How can your family tame the beast or at least beat it this time? Plan. Plan. Plan.

> **CARE TIP:** Remember that "nursing home care" can include short-term rehabilitation and long-term care.

Never Say Never

The knee jerk reaction when I ask a client "Where will you go if you need a nursing home for therapy?" is almost always "I am *not* going into a nursing home."

Me: "I know you do not want to, but let's say you fall and need rehabilitation, where are you going to go?

Client: "I don't know" and "let's not talk about it" are the usual responses.

Under most circumstances, I am a proponent of prolonged home living. The variety of options available can allow a family to care for aging and disabled loved ones at home. The means to secure those care options is a matter of strategic planning and creative combinations of support.

When I discuss nursing home care, it is most often within the context of skilled nursing and rehabilitation. The reality is: most people enter a nursing home for short- and long-term stays because of a medical situation. They experience significant enough functional, mobility, or cognitive losses that a nursing home is the most appropriate level of care.

By definition one cannot predict or control a medical crisis. However, there are some things about aging that have a high probability of occurring. One can assume those things will occur, even to his/her family. For example, as one ages the likelihood of accident or injury increases due to losses in mobility and decreases in hearing and vision.

The most common accident or injury for an older adult is a fall that results in a broken bone. The most common injury after a fall is a hip fracture. According to the National Institute of Health, one in three people over the age of 65 fall per year resulting in over 300,000 hospital admissions for hip fractures alone.[1] However, in 2004, 1.8 million people over the age of 65 fell and were treated in the emergency room. Of those people, 133,000 were admitted to the hospital for fall related complications other than a fracture. Falls are a real threat to a senior's ability to age at home.

In truth, there are many reasons loved ones have nursing home stays; however; one of the more common reasons for hospital admissions among older adults is a fall and resultant fracture. Beyond the obvious fact that a fall and fracture *could* happen is the likelihood that it *will* happen. Thirty-three percent of people age 65 and older experience a fall that results in a fracture. The number of people who fall is probably more, as many older adults hide falls from their caregivers. Seniors fear revealing a need for help and opening themselves to moving into a nursing home.

I fully appreciate your concerns about moving into a nursing home for any length of time. I consider the generational concerns and what nursing centers and convalescent homes meant during your younger years. I understand the loss of independence moving into a facility implies. The suggestion that nursing homes are "full of sick people" is a frequently expressed concern.

One of my clients, an elderly widow, was upset about her previous nursing and rehabilitation experience and was adamant about not returning. She reported the care received at the facility was okay, but the view from her room was directly into a neighboring cemetery. While that is obviously poor planning on the builder's part, I appreciate the meaning that she did not state aloud. For many older adults, being in a nursing home indicates an end of life altogether or, at the very least, an end of the quality of life to which they are accustomed.

Not many in the younger generation can truly relate to that. How does it feel to be over 90 years old? To have lost basic abilities like driving and self care. What conversations must one have with oneself when spouses, friends, siblings, and even adult children have already been lost?

I appreciate the challenges older adults face. Further, I understand their desire to maintain a tight grasp on their remaining independence. So, when a person states a disinterest in talking about nursing home care, I take my own advice. I simply plant the seed. I plant the seed that planning is necessary and provide them with the tools and information they need to connect with a quality nursing home provider when they need it for short- or long-term care. That is the most a wise caregiver can do.

Before you lose your taste for this topic, recall my earlier instruction about the continuum of care which illustrated the fact that nursing home care includes short-term rehabilitation and long-term care. Not every nursing home stay is a long-term experience. Any conversations with your loved one about nursing home care should clearly distinguish the length of time and purpose of seeking the care. Some people stay for a few weeks of therapy or for a particular drug regimen.

A nursing home setting is in-patient, meaning it could be "home" for three weeks or three months. Regardless of the length of time you stay there, the ultimate goal is to be satisfied, well cared for, and to have peace of mind in the experience. *The best way to achieve this goal is to plan even if you never want to live in a facility.* To paraphrase an old saying, it is better to have the preparation and not use it than to need it and not have it.

Remember our devoted Mrs. Johnson. Does avoiding this common loss of control illustrated in the introductory scenario about her situation motivate you to plan for nursing home care? If you are not motivated to plan, know this: as you and your loved ones age or lose abilities, the likelihood of needing nursing and rehabilitation increases. If you have not planned, you will face choosing nursing home care in the same crisis role as "Mrs. Johnson." It's your choice.

How to Prepare Well

What practical steps should your family take to prepare? The basic first steps include the following:

1). Understand what you are seeking in a nursing home stay.

Has your loved one had an accident or injury that requires a specific skill to address the problem? Alternatively, are you simply seeking a nursing home for long-term supervision needs? Hip replacements and general weakness related to dealing with pneumonia are common occurrences in nursing homes. Almost any licensed nursing and rehabilitation center *should* be able to provide appropriate nursing and rehabilitation care. With that said, therapists and nurses come with a variety of clinical experiences and training. For this reason, the effectiveness of nursing care and physical challenges and rigor of a therapy program can vary greatly.

For example, most every therapy gym should have parallel bars, which therapists can use while retraining a person's balance and walking. However, some therapy areas have very little equipment to help your therapists deliver a dynamic treatment program. Regardless of the amount of equipment in a therapy department or the title of the therapist, you should feel challenged in the therapy regimen whether your diagnosis is basic or complex.

What if you have other conditions or specialized medical needs? These needs may include deafness, dementia, obesity, or other complex medical diagnoses. For example, not every facility can or will accept a patient who is morbidly obese due to the specialized equipment needed to care for that person. An obese person may need a special bed, special mechanical lift machine to move in and out of the bed (a Hoyer lift), a special wheelchair, and a walker that will support his/her weight, to name a few equipment needs.

If the facility admits a patient who is obese, they are not only agreeing to accept that person's insurance as payment. The facility is also agreeing to care for that person in the same way they should care for anyone else. The size of a patient is not an excuse for inadequate care.

2). Visit several nursing homes in your local area before you need that level of care. The first visit to any nursing home can be overwhelming. Proper advanced planning offers the luxury of going home after a nursing home tour, thinking it over, and feeling more confident that because of your efforts you will choose the best facility for your loved one.

No matter how grand the nursing home building and grounds, families must ensure the facility is worthy of entrusting the well-being of their loved one. Peace of mind is worth a 30-minute visit to a nursing home, even if that visit occurs during a lunch hour. Getting there is the hardest part. I know you do not want to consider it. I know you do not want to think about it. I also know you want the best quality of care possible for yourself and/or your loved one.

There are several theories on conquering fears. On theory is to jump right in and face the fear head-on to shock the senses. The other theories encourage gradual desensitization. To translate this into planning for nursing homes, you can throw yourself into the process of visiting and touring or you can take the more measured approach. You can simply drive by several facilities, progress yourself to pulling into the parking lot, and then one day (hopefully before you need the care) you might just walk-in and take a tour. Take inventory of your apprehensions about nursing homes and rehabilitation facilities and then pick a method and *"get 'er done."*

Finding quality of care will not happen by accident. Too often, the people I see after a nursing home experience do not plan to return to the same facility. I hope your nursing home experiences are better. Are you willing to risk a less than ideal experience? Avoiding the nursing home visits and interviews only postpones the probable (needing the care). Procrastination robs you of any chance to choose a facility on your own terms. Advanced planning for nursing home care ensures you will receive care where you prefer, not just where there is an acceptable opening.

I hear you say, "But my dad does not want to go into a nursing home." I know he does not and if you like him you probably do not *want* to put him there either. Sometimes wants do not mesh with reality. The older he gets the more likely he will need short-term rehabilitation in a skilled nursing and rehabilitation center.

How do you frame this discussion so the dreaded words "nursing home" do not end the talk before it begins? Focus on the "short-term rehabilitation." Using the words "rehabilitation center" completely changes the context of the conversation. Even the word "rehab" implies a higher level of care that is temporary. The words "nursing home" imply a long-term arrangement. If you and your family feel a long-term nursing home stay is most appropriate, perhaps you should be clear about your intentions. To be clear, I am <u>not</u> advocating the use of the word rehabilitation unless short-term rehabilitation is your sincere intention.

3). Get professional help from an impartial advocate if you are not comfortable weighing options. There are two distinct types of assistance available during nursing home care. One is administrative, the other is personalized. The administrative assistance can come from your state's Long-term Care Ombudsman Program. The Ombudsman can provide information about how a facility performed in the most recent health inspections and providing information about the complaints a facility has received. The personalized assistance comes from an experienced elder care specialist. Elder care consulting services, such as those provided by Pope Institute, add value to your family's experience. The information, resources, and personal support you receive to make informed decisions and take control of day-to-day challenges will be well worth it.

I provide assistance on an ongoing and as needed basis. For example, I help my clients find a nursing home, answer a client's "what-if" questions, check-in on a loved one in a facility, attend conferences at the facility, advocate for my client, and provide my professional guidance that is grounded in many years of experience as a nursing home professional. I help my client manage challenges and avoid crises when possible.

4). Trust but verify. While a particular facility or professional may come recommended by Aunt Betty, it does not mean that provider is the right fit for you. While standards of care should not vary, quality is a perception of each consumer. Quality depends very much on cultural expectations, medical needs, and personal preferences. While referrals from friends and family are a good place to start, you must evaluate the facility for yourself.

Many consumers are hesitant in asking questions of health care providers. They do not feel comfortable doing what is necessary to critically assess facilities. Part of this intimidation is because consumers do not have experience in this area. Consumers usually trust things are the way they appear. They keep that perception until proven otherwise. Sometimes the proof of trustworthiness comes when a family has already committed to a particular agency, professional caregiver, or health care provider.

It is much easier to change your mind initially. However, it is not impossible to change direction at any time. Your health care benefits travel with you. If one provider is not meeting your needs, considering moving to your secondary facility of choice, if in fact you have toured and critically evaluated enough facilities to have three *preferred* providers.

5). Realize long-term care is a business. Like all businesses, long-term care providers exist to serve the consumer. Ask for what you want (within reason); if you do not get it, consider going somewhere else. It is your right, privilege, and duty as a consumer to hold providers responsible for inadequate care. My one piece of advice: please be reasonable in your requests. Do not demand care that extends beyond quality into that which is purely preferential. Asking for what you want is about reasonable accommodation and meeting at least the minimum standards of care. I am not talking about demanding veal parmesan on the menu or personalized attention that requires everyone else in the facility to wait until your requests are met.

I believe most nursing home providers want satisfied customer-patients. Work with your nursing home provider to achieve that end. If you find that your satisfaction is not their priority, perhaps you should consider moving your money, your health benefits, and your loved one to a facility that is willing and able to meet your expectations.

6). View yourself as a consumer. Customer satisfaction is the key to successful business. So why are nursing homes continuing to prosper financially while the average consumer dreads the idea of even a short-term stay? Do you view yourself as a "consumer" of health care? Why are health care consumer expectations and actions of accountability different from other goods and services?

Let's say you went to dinner at a nice restaurant. Maybe a friend recommended the restaurant or maybe you just drove by and thought it looked like a good place to eat. The host is welcoming, seats you at a table, and you feel good about the selection. Upon receiving your meal, you realize it is not what you expected. In fact, it looks nothing like what was on the menu. You inform the waiter that your food is not up to par. He then tells you the restaurant is short staffed, the cook is having a bad day, and they are doing their best. Therefore, under the circumstances, he cannot fix your meal, nor can he adjust your dinner bill.

Would you continue to eat the unappetizing meal? Would you accept a mere apology or expect some accommodations? How long would it take you to speak with a manager and request a refund or discount? Would you consider filing a formal complaint or writing an appropriate criticism of the restaurant? While eating at a fine restaurant differs from a nursing home experience, and not just in the food department, the fact is you are a consumer in both settings. I wonder if health care consumers would be stronger advocates for quality of care if they were paying for the care out-of-pocket like in the restaurant. Your meal and your health care will not get better if you do not speak up about shortcomings in the system. If you will buy mediocrity, what is their incentive for improvement?

7). Hope for the best, but have a plan B & a plan C. Most seniors would rather live the rest of their lives at home without interruption. There is truly no place like home. When I coach caregivers about her parent's apprehension about nursing homes, I remind clients of what convalescent homes were like during her parents' and grandparents' younger years. They were warehouses for people with misdiagnosed mental illness; those abandoned by their families, a catch all for miscellaneous social and medical problems, and they involved a mix of "treatment" interventions that occasionally show up in horror movies. It is no wonder seniors view a nursing home as nothing to seek!

While most seniors want to age at home forever and never go into a nursing home, the reality is nursing home care may be required after a fall or injury. Because of injury, many people require nursing home care for short-term rehabilitation—occupational and physical therapy. Over eight million people each year experience nursing home and home health care. Of those in nursing homes, 1.6 million remain in the facility for an extended stay.[2]

How many of those eight million people do you think actually planned to receive home health care or enter a nursing home for any length of time? Further, how many of that 1.6 million chose that facility before they needed nursing home care? I would submit to you that most of the millions who receive long-term care services do *not* develop a long-term care plan. People may plan for the financial aspect of needing nursing home care, by having insurance. Yet many more do not plan for the qualitative part of nursing home care. The qualitative aspect is *where* those insurance benefits are utilized.

While nursing home care is not the topic of choice, neglecting the conversation with one's family can be costly in terms of quality of care and overall satisfaction.

How to Choose a Good Home

The most effective tool in your quest for a good nursing home is the effort you place in planning for nursing home care. This includes visiting multiple facilities on multiple occasions. The multiple visits allow you to see the physical, social, and cultural environment in which one will reside.

I will say it again; multiple facilities and multiple visits is the only way to gauge the real culture of a facility. By *culture* I mean the overall feeling and tone of the facility. Culture includes the emotional warmth of interactions between the staff and the residents as well as the interaction between staff members and management.

After working in nursing homes for many years in various regions of the U.S., I can assure you that corporate culture is important. Staff interpersonal relationships and management/staff relationships have a measurable influence on the emotional health of a facility. It is part of the reason companies in health care and many other industries perform regular staff satisfaction surveys. I have seen it time and again;

happy, accountable, and appreciated staff make loving and kind caregivers.

A facility's emotional health and a clean physical environment are aspects that families should look for when touring and visiting a prospective facility. The absence of these features is a potential deal breaker in my opinion. What in particular are features on which families should not settle? Among the top priorities are:

1). A clean physical environment

Some nursing home entries could double for the lobby of a 5-star hotel. Grandeur does not make a facility good at its purpose of caring for people. While plush is nice, clean is mandatory. If you smell urine or other easily manageable odors, let your nose lead you out the door! In an age of highly effective cleaning chemicals and sanitization products, odor is inexcusable. Period.

Some facilities allow odor to permeate their hallways. I have entered nursing homes that are malodorous, yet full of patients and everyone seemed to be okay with it. Odor is not okay. A notable and ongoing presence of odor indicates either the residents are not cleaned well and/or the facility itself is not well cleaned.

Speaking of cleanliness, I recall observing a nurse aide during his morning routine with patients. He had a jolly attitude while he worked with a brain injured man. He gave the person a sponge bath in the bed which took no more than 5 minutes. This time included the turning of the patient, wringing of the towel, and the washing of this person. He brushed the gentleman's hair and concluded the grooming session.

I thought, *"that is the quickest bath I have ever seen!"* As the aide went about fixing the bed and straightening up the patient's room, I could not help myself. I got a clean towel from the patient's bathroom and proceeded to clean his ears, which were filthy, and washed his eyebrows and nose as best I could. His eyebrows and nose were coated with what resembled the white filmy substance that covers newborn babies.

I could not believe another human being could consider someone clean after a cursory five minute sponge bath. It was not the amount of time that was at issue, it was the lack of effort and attention paid to areas that obviously needed washing.

Judging by the results of closer inspection, this person had not received a thorough washing in a long-time. Since that day, I have always paid attention to the ears, eyebrows, and hairline of residents. Skin accumulates if you have a dermatological condition such as seborrheic dermatitis, eczema, or psoriasis. Barring a skin condition, accumulation of dead skin cells is more likely to occur if one is not washed and moisturized well. It is not acceptable.

2). Lack of staff warmth toward visitors and residents

To be sure, there are bad apples in every bunch. There are bound to be staff that does not fit the mold of a "caregiver." That is not an excuse. It is simply the reality of any workplace. The test of nursing home management is to rid the facility of the bad influences, preferably before they ruin the entire staff and the reputation of a facility.

Families should look for caring and respectful interactions between staff and the residents. If you visit a facility and observe general behavior that departs from that standard, I would move on and keep looking.

The front line staff in a nursing home has one of the toughest and most important jobs in the facility. Sometimes life outside of the facility can influence a professional's mood. A particularly difficult resident can make your day harder. A co-worker calling in sick can double a work load. Any of these things can make an ordinarily mild mannered person a little irritable.

The test of professionalism is to keep oneself firmly in contact with it no matter the circumstances that present a challenge. There are plenty of challenges with working in long-term care. Some managers are condescending and rude. Some residents in nursing homes are confused or demented or simply do not want to be there, and demonstrate their frustration toward the staff. It is each professional's responsibility to not pass on that frustration to the residents under their charge.

3). Unhappy residents and staff

If the people who already live in a facility do not seem pleased in their decision, I'd take the hint straightaway. Your experience may not be that different. If the staff appears unhappy or preoccupied with events outside of the facility or seem disconnected from their purpose for being there (caregiving), it is an indicator of the lack of attention to care.

You may be able to talk with the staff to get their insider's perception of the facility. Frustrated staff will be more than happy to provide information. If an administrator is a strict enforcer of timeliness and accountability, resentment may color the feedback you receive and can bias the information from staff.

By talking with staff members, you are seeking *balanced* information. You may ask what they like about working at the facility. Ask when was the last time they had to work short-staffed. Ask if they placed their loved one in the facility what would be their primary concern. Ask what they think the facility could improve to make the staff happier and what steps the facility could take to improve resident care. As with all human communication, the non-verbal cues can be more revealing than verbal responses. Scoffs, laughs, tsks, rolled eyes, shrugs, and shaking heads are definite points of clarification.

The answers you receive give an idea of how people on the inside view the facility. Of course you have to consider the source and evaluate the answers for transparency. Responses that are flattering and vague may be untrue or protective. On the other hand, responses about management attempts to enforce accountability may indicate strong and diligent managers. Either way, it does not hurt to ask the questions and gauge the manner in which the answers are given. You may get a more honest response if the question is posed without a witness.

Here is a suggestion, if you find a visitor (family member) in the facility or parking lot, talk with her about her perception of the nursing home. Ask her about the quality of care she has received. Ask her which staff does a good job and which ones she feels could use a little guidance. Ask about how her concerns have been managed. Also ask what she has heard about the facility. Basically, ask the family member about the good, bad, and the ugly. You may find some relevant information that you otherwise would not get.

4). Unprofessional behavior

Have you ever worked in an office environment where you might as well have been standing on a street corner? Open displays of loud, rude, and generally unprofessional behavior should not be expected or accepted. In the nursing home environment, employees are basically working in the shared home of the residents of the facility. If you find overt displays of unprofessionalism in the hallways, dining rooms, and other common areas, chances are that type of behavior is generally accepted and you can expect more of the same.

Lest I appear unfair, allow me to say I understand the need for energized and fun work environments. I have shared many laughs with co-workers about a pre-scholar's first dance recital, a spouse's failed attempt at fixing a household issue, or a cooking mishap that defies imagination. The reality is life lived to the fullest is fun and is at times downright hilarious! Sometimes you want to share those laughs with your friends at work-at the appropriate time and in an appropriate manner. There is a clear distinction between fun and unprofessional. Most professionals do not need a flashlight to find that line.

5). It just doesn't feel right!

If you visit 50 nursing homes, and you probably won't, but if you did, you will find few general differences. The facilities either have "it" or they do not. I liken assessing nursing homes to eating liver; either you like it or you don't! I mean no offense to nursing homes or liver. If you've eaten liver, you know what I mean. A non-committal assessment like "it was ok" basically means at best I would prefer something else.

Trust your instincts. If the facility does not feel right, do not second guess. If you perceive the sales pitch shines brighter than what you observe, move on. During your multiple visits (hint, hint), decide with your gut. *Do not* talk yourself into an ill fitting relationship.

What happens with families who settle for "it was okay?" It looks something like this: visiting frequently if not every day to "just make sure everything is all right," keeping a close watch on everything and everyone you observe, and going home after each visit feeling insecure and on pins and needles because you cannot be at the facility 24/7.

Give yourself a break! There are over 14,000 nursing homes in the United States. Most of them do not run at one hundred percent occupancy. This means there is usually a bed available in one of the three nursing homes or skilled nursing facilities that you prefer. Your nursing home experience should be a collaborative effort between your family and the facility you choose. Your hyper-vigilance indicates a discomfort and breakdown in collaboration. If you do your homework, you would find an ideal facility before you need short- or long-term nursing home care. The only way to get the desirable total care environment you want is to do the homework *now*. By front loading your efforts, you will not spend hours later as a watch guard trying to make lemonade out of lemons. Do not settle for less.

With these basic guidelines in mind, how do you go about completing your multiple visits to multiple facilities? The easy answer is you give a call and tell the facility you are interested in touring. Take along your nursing home checklist which is available by emailing lifebydesign@popeinstitute.com.

Since you are selecting a facility in advance of needing the care, you can afford to be more critical. Now is the ideal time to put on your inspector's cap.   Be courteous; be critical (not necessarily aloud). Document what you observe as you complete your tours and multiple visits.

Who's Driving This Ship?

As previously stated, health care is a business as are the various services included within the health care industry.   Since we live in a capitalistic society, we all recognize that businesses drive our economy. The success of these businesses also affect the stability of the job market on which working people depend, as do unemployed people who receive benefits from programs funded by payroll taxes. There are many reasons companies decide to organize in a "for-profit" or not-for profit structure.   There is no inherent problem with either choice.   The organizational focus rather than the organizational structure of a company will affect quality of care. This is true for short- and long-term care facilities.

The reality is, regardless of a business's "for profit" or "not-for-profit" status, the company has to actually make a profit in order to keep operating A not-for-profit company that does not make a profit may find itself closing its doors, no matter how noble its mission. With that said, profit should never take precedent over care. The problem occurs when a company's perspective on profit leads to negative consequences for quality of care.

For example, in the summer of 2007, Dr. David Barton Smith, a Temple University professor and his research team, released an unsettling research report about race, poverty, and nursing home care. An article about the research findings appeared in the <u>St. Louis Post Dispatch</u>. An interviewee in the article mentioned that the troubled nursing homes "would like to provide quality care but just can't afford to." My published editorial in response to that comment highlighted an important concept; it is unacceptable for any care provider to claim a desire to provide quality care but an inability to do so for financial reasons. While Medicaid reimburses facilities a small amount compared to what the facilities charge for their services, the facilities are obviously making enough money to remain in operation. Profit is good and necessary, but quality of care is not optional; it is the standard.

A trend in health care that reflects the need for this principle is the purchasing of nursing homes by large private equity firms. The private equity firm will purchase a nursing home provider and turn the company around to be more profitable. The problem is that some of the private equity firms changed the facilities operations in a manner that made them forty-one percent more profitable than the average nursing home.[3] Again the problem is not the profit, however, at the same time profits increased, reportedly, the quality of care dropped and complaints and health violations increased.[4] The <u>New York Times</u> broke the story which resulted in Senator Hillary Rodham Clinton calling for a congressional investigation of the private equity firms and their previous and planned nursing home purchases.

How prevalent is this issue? According to the <u>New York Times</u> as of fall 2007, private equity firms controlled over 200,000 nursing home beds and over 14,000 other homes. Depending on the outcome of the investigations, the number of nursing home purchases could increase because the opportunity to be more profitable than average is pretty attractive for any business. This illustration does not mean all private equity firms have practices that compromise quality of care. Yet, the <u>New York Times</u>' report does highlight the fact that consumers may want to inquire about ownership of a long-term care facility.

How can you find out if your nursing home or senior housing complex is owned by a private equity firm? In evaluating ownership of a senior living home, especially a nursing home, it is important to know the focus and history of the company. Patterns of cutting staff; nurses in particular, and the pattern of cutting programs and quality of life activities require further investigation. If you ask a facility administrator, you may not get a clear answer about the number of staff cuts. The facility's activities director or social services director would also know about changes in programs. During your tours and multiple visits, you can inquire about program changes, and may become privy to the result of such changes through conversations with the staff and residents.

Touring and Interviewing Nursing Homes

This process is just that, an interview. You are interviewing candidate facilities to care for your loved one or yourself. It is a serious job and you are doing the hiring. Call to schedule an appointment or just walk-in one day, which I recommend with subsequent visits. The nursing home Administrator (manager) or the Director of Admissions (marketer) will lead a guided tour of the facility.

I have spent many years working in nursing homes as a therapist; years spent working with Administrators and Admissions Directors. After time spent functioning as an Administrator-in-Training and as an Interim Director of Admissions and Marketing, I fully understand the role and function of each of these professionals.

As you would expect, administrators and marketers typically make great first impressions. After all, when was the last time you bought a product from a slouchy salesperson? Administrators can set the tone for a well-organized facility and instill an expectation of high quality care. However, do not feel inclined to sign an admissions contract based solely on your impression of the administration. Residents will have limited direct contact with this level of management in daily life at the facility.

The nurses and nurse's aides deliver the bulk of direct care to nursing home residents. As a result, the Director of Nursing (DON) and the Assistant Director(s) of Nursing (ADONs) are an important part of the management team. A family should meet those professionals during tours and visits.

Meeting with the administrator and the nursing management staff can give you an idea of the management style in the facility and customer service style of managing your concerns. Meeting with or evaluating the staff will provide more information. This includes tone of voice when speaking with residents and the overall staff professionalism. The culture of the facility itself will give an indication as to how daily operations reflect the image cast by administration and the facility's grandeur.

If possible, schedule a couple of visits for 30 minutes before and during a mealtime to observe how staff responds under stress. Mealtime in nursing homes can be hectic depending on the structure and logistics of meal delivery. Observe how staff deals with stress and caring for dependent residents. Does the meal service have a pleasant and calm undertone, or is it chaotic and rushed? Observe how staff copes with residents who require coaxing or a greater amount of physical assistance to eat. Observe if there is a sense of compassionate engagement that respects the individuality of each person or simply work performance in feeding residents.

During mealtime, you have the advantage of observing several staff members at once. Further, if you visit at several meal times (breakfast, lunch, or dinner) you are likely to see a variety of caregivers who you otherwise may not.

Nursing homes, like any work place, have employees with varying levels of commitment and skills to meet the essential challenges of the job. Your job is to take every measure to understand what you need, search for facilities that meet your needs, and know how to hold providers accountable including seeking advocacy to get good care or moving to your secondary facility of choice.

Cultural Considerations

If your loved one is deaf and uses sign language, communication with staff could be limited. How will issues of pain be clearly communicated, for example? How will he describe the location of the pain, the severity of the pain, the duration of the pain, when it started, when it is worse, and what makes it better? Alternatively, does your loved one have ethnic or cultural practices that influence their quality of life?

If your family is managing these special needs, it is important to seek assistance from an experienced elder care specialist who can appreciate the multicultural perspectives that may otherwise be overlooked.

Getting Reasonable Accommodations

What types of accommodations is a family likely to want? For practical purposes, almost everything in a nursing home is scheduled. There are waking times, medication times, meal times, therapy times, and organized recreational activities. A couple of common questions that arise when the nursing home schedule does not mesh well with a patient's schedule include:

1). If I prefer to rise late can I do so without the possibility of missing meals or other aspects of my care, such as scheduled showers? If so, what is the method of communicating agreed upon accommodations to the staff that create and carry out the schedule on a day-to-day basis? What is the course of action if accommodations are not honored on a consistent basis?

2). How are roommates assigned and can I have some input into who is my roommate? Seek clarification on the policy for room assignments. NOTE: federal   housing   regulations   restrict   broad   based accommodations of cultural preferences based on race, religion, and ethnicity as such "accommodations" unfairly hinder the quality of life of others.

3). Some nursing homes have large rooms that four residents share. If you are in a semi-private, room with more than two roommates and do not prefer that arrangement, talk with the administrator or social services director. Inform them that when a room with only two beds becomes available you would like the opportunity to move. Remember to check-in with the social services department periodically as a friendly reminder of your request.

With diligence, commitment, and accountability, within 60 days of starting the process you should be able to find two to three skilled nursing and rehabilitation centers (nursing homes) that you like. The goal is to feel comfortable entrusting your care or the care of a loved one. I hear you say, "That sounds like a lot of work." The work you complete now will save time and stress when you need the nursing home level of care. If you find your commitment waning, consider what is hindering your progress. Evaluate your views on nursing homes. Are your emotions causing you to stumble in the planning process? Alternatively, are you motivated to plan but simply need guidance on getting started? Do you need an accountability partner to help you finish the planning process?

Tools for Nursing Home Selection

A resource of which consumers should be aware is "Nursing Home Compare," the online Medicare nursing home comparison tool. The nursing home compare tool is an online compilation of nursing homes that are Medicare and Medicaid certified. The online tool provides information about the number of beds, if the facility is not-for-profit or for-profit, the date of the last state health survey inspection, and much more.

Nursing Home Compare also provides consumers with detailed information about what it calls quality measures. The nineteen Nursing Home Compare quality measures include percentages of patients with pain, percentage of patients with bedsores, and percentage of patients with other generally undesirable secondary health related conditions.

The Nursing Home Compare information can be a good starting point to find facilities in a 500-mile radius of your home. There are no hard and fast rules about distance between your home and a nursing home. I advise families to choose a travel distance that they find acceptable for regular visits. A ten- to fifteen-mile radius is a reasonable distance to travel for visits, but many factors may cause you to exceed that recommendation. When deciding on a distance, consider when you are most likely to visit your loved one--weekends only or weekdays regularly. If you visit on weekdays, consider the traffic patterns in the direction of travel. For example, if you live in the Atlanta metro area, you may want to reconsider weekday evening visits to the city, unless you have time to spend on the highway.

Regular visits are important for your loved one to feel connected and for you to have peace of mind. If you feel you must be at the facility at all times to ensure good care, you are in the wrong facility. If nothing near your home gives you that home-away-from-home feeling and you are concerned about your loved one's safety, increase your search radius. This may mean having to travel a little farther (within reason) to get the care you want. Ask yourself this question: "Is it more important to find the facility that feels like "home," gives me peace of mind, and provides the care I want, or one that is extra convenient for traveling?" Realize you may not find what you seek in your immediate area and adjust accordingly.

> **CARE TIP**: An elder care specialist can help you choose local nursing homes when you want personalized guidance rather than administrative support. A consultant can also help you monitor a loved one in another state.

Upon choosing a facility, verify health survey information with your state or local Long-term Care Ombudsman Program. Every state has a long-term care ombudsman and many metropolitan areas have local ombudsman programs.

In evaluating whether your family needs an elder care specialist or a long-term care ombudsman, I would suggest the two services are *complementary* and not interchangeable. The long-term care ombudsman has access to current administrative health survey and complaint information. A qualified elder care specialist, such as those available at Pope Institute, will help with one-to-one guidance about long term care planning, facilitate regular and routine visits to monitor a loved one's status (especially when out of state), and can function as a personal family advocate for day-to-day coordination of care needs and managing crises. Not all elder care specialists are the same. A qualified elder care specialist with broad experience in the health care system can also guide your family throughout the continuum of care including and beyond the nursing home setting.

You Should Know

A word of caution when considering the information from Nursing Home Compare or the state survey; consider the surveyors observe the facility for a relatively short amount of time. Most surveys last a week or less. In addition, many surveys are announced to the facility before hand. Therefore, the facility has the opportunity to get things in shape for the sake of compliance. Further, during "surprise" surveys, the element of surprise is lost the minute surveyors announce who they are and the staff is alerted to their presence. Moreover, several factors can affect the thoroughness of a survey including the relationship with administration, the critical eye of the surveyor, and acceptance of management stated plans of correction to resolve noted problems, which can avoid a record of an identified problem.

Even a facility with zero deficits can have serious problems with quality of care. With that said, the survey information is better than nothing or relying on facility reported information, but you have to critically evaluate the facility yourself and seek support from a qualified elder care specialist when needed. While survey data is good to have, it should not be your sole source of objective information.

Getting What You Bought

When you need to use one of the ideal nursing home facilities, how do you ensure quality of care when you get there? It is true that you should not feel your presence at the home 24/7 is the only reason your loved one gets good care. However, most facilities perform better with a little accountability. That accountability can come from your family or from a hired advocate if you have real concerns or simply want an experienced set of eyes and ears.

The first step in getting good care is to know your patient rights and know how those rights should affect the care you receive. In 1997, President Bill Clinton appointed a health commission to formulate standards of quality care. Out of that Presidential commission, the patient's bill of rights was adopted.

Patients' Rights in brief are:

- The Right to Information. Patients have the right to receive accurate and easy to understand information to assist in evaluating options for services, care providers, and health coverage.

- The Right to Choose. Patients have the right to a choice of what professional caregiver works with you. This includes access to specialists such as an obstetrician and gynecologist, and care for complex medical situations, and chronic diseases.

- Access to Emergency Services. Patients have the right to receive emergency health services (ER) at the time of need at the nearest appropriate location. This patient right sets guidelines as to under what circumstance and to what extent your health plan can regulate emergency health care services.

- Being a Full Partner in Health Care Decisions. Patients are encouraged to be active participants in all decisions about their care. Consumers who are unable to participate in treatment decisions have the right to be represented by parents, guardians, family members, or other conservators. A health care professional should not be limited by written or implied restrictions that prevent discussion of medically necessary treatment options. This is true even if the options are not available through the health care professional's employer.

- Care without Discrimination. Patients should be afforded the rights to appropriate health care services throughout the continuum of care with out regard to race, ethnicity, religion, nationality, age, gender, or current or probably mental or physical handicap, or ability to pay.

- The Right to Privacy. Patients have the right to communicate personal and confidential information to their doctor, nurses, and other health care practitioners with the expectation that their individually identifiable health care information will be protected. Patients also have the right to review and copy their own medical records and request amendments to their records.

- The Right to Speedy Complaint Resolution. Patients have the right to a fair and efficient process for resolving differences with their health plans, health care providers, and the institutions that serve them, including a rigorous system of internal review and an independent system of external review.

- You should find pre-established grievance processes available to your family. This may include written forms that a family can complete. In filing a complaint, families should become privy to the chain of command and organization structure through which a complaint may travel.

- Taking on New Responsibilities. Patients are expected to assume individual responsibility for their care including observing healthy lifestyle habits, participating in preventative health measures, and seeking timely medical treatment.

Federal Law has established additional rights specific to nursing home residents and these rights include:

Respect: You have the right to be treated with dignity and respect. One of the primary annoyances is to observe facility caregivers treat an older adult like a cute child. Another is poor humor that plays into an elderly person's concerns which results in them getting agitated. Those who are sensitive to the rule of respect make every attempt to avoid using poor humor or calling older adults endearing monikers without their consent.

Services and Fees: You must be informed in writing about services and fees before you enter the nursing home. During the interview phase, you will ask for and should receive the service fee information. You can also ask for a sample of any entrance contract you will have to sign. The entrance contract should highlight services, fees, and billing practices.

Money: You have the right to manage your own money or to choose someone else you trust to manage money for you. Income you receive from Social Security that is due to the facility can be paid directly from you or a designated family member. The Social Security check does not have to be signed over to a facility. Your family can write a check payable to the facility. Keep in mind; you are ultimately responsible for any charges related to your care. These charges include Medicare co-pays and the Medicaid spend-down (see Chapter Five). If you or a family member squanders the Social Security income, you may face collection activity, and other financial and legal problems related to the delinquent bill. The facility can also discharge you for not paying in a timely fashion.

Privacy: You have the right to privacy. You have the right to keep and use your personal belongings and property with you. This is true as long as it does not interfere with the rights, health, or safety of other residents.

Medical Care: You have the right to be informed about your medical condition, medications, and to see your own doctor. You also have the right to refuse medications and treatments. That means you and your designated family members have a right to pose questions and receive complete and consumer friendly explanations.

What are some real world applications to the nursing home patient rights? Examples of patient right challenges include:

1). Making your own schedule including rising, eating, and participating in activities.

2). You have the right to live in an environment that is free from harassment, free from abuse, and free from retaliation for complaining about the presence of harassment or abuse.

3). Being discharged from a nursing home for issues other than those allowed by law, which include:

- Your presence of actions endanger the welfare, health and safety of yourself or others

- It is no longer medically appropriate for you to remain in a nursing home due to significant health improvement or significant health declines

- The nursing home has not been paid for services you received

- The nursing home closes

Discharges or transfers from a nursing home for reasons other than those provided for by law are prohibited.

4). Your health information should only be shared with staff working directly on your case. Further, only those family members you have authorized in writing should receive information about your health and medical care. This includes access to your medical record and the ability to limit who is informed of your current medical status. Everyone who has visited a doctor or filled a prescription within the last several years has signed a HIPAA (Health Insurance Portability and Accountability Act) form.

The government requires every health care provider to inform you of their HIPAA policy. The policy explains how the health care provider will use and disclose your personal identifying information. This includes any information that can identify you individually and any past, current, or future health information that is linked to you directly.

Common Problems and Complaints

They only gave me two days to get her ready to go home.

Nursing homes are required by law to give at least three days notice of a discharge related to progress or the lack thereof. The facility has several meetings where progress is discussed. The number of meetings you have depends on how long you stay at a skilled nursing and rehabilitation center. You should have at least one family meeting within the first couple of weeks to talk with all the therapists and health professionals. This meeting will cover therapy goals, your loved one's status, and an estimate of how much treatment may be appropriate.

The facility also has a weekly administrative meeting-- Medicare Utilization meeting. The facility nurses, discharge planners, and therapists discuss the use of your Medicare benefits. This is the meeting where discharges for the upcoming days or coming week are discussed. I would encourage families to talk regularly with the therapists to monitor when a discharge may be recommended.

A projected discharge in ten days could shrink to four days with significant progress or the lack of it. If you have a need for skilled nursing care (e.g., for a wound), you may be able to remain in a skilled nursing facility without therapy services. After the facility's weekly Medicare Utilization meeting, the discharge planner will notify your family by issuing a written three-day notice of discharge. If you do not receive that notice at least three days before a discharge, you should inform your state's long-term care ombudsman. The ombudsman may be able to halt a discharge if appropriate.

He is not compliant and the facility wants to discharge him.

Sometimes a facility will threaten to seek a discharge if the family does not pursue guardianship. For example, a facility wants a caregiver to seek legal guardianship for a loved one so the caregiver can "force" the patient to be compliant. Unfortunately, some patients have a history of mental illness and a history of violence including demonstrating physical aggression against nursing home workers. The award of guardianship depends on the court finding a person incompetent to make sound decisions. This may require a trial if the patient objects to the guardianship request.

Even if a guardianship is awarded and the guardian wants and tells the patient to comply with treatment procedures or a medication regimen, it may be difficult to force compliance. It may also cause a multitude of issues for the facility to force a patient to participate in treatments.

A patient has the right to refuse treatment. Refusing to take medication, refusing to take a bath, and refusing to allow certain procedures are not *necessarily* a reason to transfer a patient to another facility. If the patient is becoming a danger to himself or herself or someone else in the facility, a nursing home has every right to seek a transfer to another facility. If however it is simply a matter of refusing treatment, a patient has every right to do so.

The best advice is to talk with an elder law attorney about which type of legal document (see Chapter Eight) would be most appropriate for your situation.

The food here is bad

This has to be one of the most common complaints about nursing homes. If you live in a 100-bed nursing home, the cooks prepare meals for 100 dietary restrictions. Some patients have low sodium requirements, dietary fat restrictions, some have low sugar requirements, and some have no restrictions at all. In the health care environment, the possible exceptions being the hospital and assisted living settings, bland for everyone is safe. With the advent of products that taste like the real thing but without the associated health risks, food in nursing homes should be improving. You can get fake butter spread and salt that make mashed potatoes taste almost like restaurant style.

If you are dissatisfied with the food, inform your administrator and add some constructive ideas to the suggestion box. The cooks in the nursing home kitchen are rarely trained chefs unless they work in an upscale facility or a nursing home that realizes good food is a great way to warm the hearts of its residents. Here's a suggestion, ask to sample the food during your tours and visits.

Some residents have family members deliver home cooked meals daily because they do not like the food. Others have take-out delivered to the nursing home.

Despite the culinary blandness of nursing home food, spoiled, rotten, or stale food is not acceptable and should be reported to your state's department of health.

They wake me at 5 am to get blood

Sometimes a nursing home will use an outside agency to perform blood draws for lab tests. Realize under certain circumstances it may be necessary to get a blood sample before your eat anything. If waking at 5 am does not work well for your internal clock, I would talk with the nursing staff to see if they can come to you later in their rounds, which may give you more time to rest.

However, there are many times orders for bloods samples are written with no end date. The doctor may want a particular blood test completed daily. Literally, there are instances where the doctor tells the patient the labs are fine and he is no longer concerned, yet along comes a lab tech to draw blood. If you question the need to continue with daily blood draws, ask the nurse to confirm that need with your doctor. It may be that the physician order to discontinue the blood samples was never written or communicated.

They keep losing my stuff

It is amazing how many dentures, hearing aids, and random articles of clothing are misplaced in nursing homes. Like a moth to a flame, hearing aids and dentures are attracted to bed linens that are bound for the laundry. While the hearing aid may not survive the washing, it may also never find its rightful owner if it is not marked with a name. Here is a piece of advice that will serve you well in trying to take home everything you brought with you; if you want to keep it, put your name on it using an indelible method. Your audiologist or the hearing aid store can etch your name onto the hearing aid. Your dentists can do the same for all sets of your dentures. The same can be done for your eyeglasses.

Upon entering the nursing home, the admissions department will instruct you to label all items of clothing with a permanent marker. Take them literally; label *everything*, including family furniture and electronics.

Familiarize yourself with the location of the lost and found. Some items are returned to the nurse's station adjacent to where it is found. Some items are returned to the administrator, to the Director of Nursing, or even to the Admission's Department. The facility may reimburse you for items that are lost or misplaced because of staff actions.

I keep doing the same thing in therapy

Several factors can contribute to the challenge and effectiveness of a therapy program. I have heard from families more frequently than I prefer that they did not feel challenged in a nursing home therapy program. Some families report they did not stand the entire time at a rehabilitation center. Others complete the same arm cycle, leg cycle, and marching in place exercises. Still others sit in the therapy gym with three other patients as one therapist attempts to alternate between sessions with each of them. This is certainly not acceptable or adequate rehabilitation.

If you are in a facility for rehabilitation, there are cases where time is of the essence for achieving adequate recovery of motor or mental function. If one facility cannot meet your rehabilitation needs, please find another that can provide a challenging and appropriate rehabilitation program. You may ask during your tours and visits if you can observe the therapy department (in the gym). As a therapist, I know that it may be difficult to know what to look for. In brief, if all you observed were the carryout of activity with little instruction, a gym full of patients and few therapists, sparse patient education, and minimal challenge, I would question the facility's priorities and ability to meet your rehabilitation needs.

If you have a question about the care you are receiving call me for assistance immediately! Time is of the essence for disabled and aged patients. A therapeutic day lost is ability lost.

I want to shower everyday, not two times per week

Nursing home regulations provide for a *minimum* number of times a resident should receive a shower within a week. An accommodation for more frequent showers is reasonable if that is your custom and preference. Inquire during your tours and interviews about the nursing home's perspective on providing staff to assist with daily showers. If the response is, "We provide showers twice per week," you should know that is a *minimum* standard. A facility can and should exceed that standard if regular showering is a quality of life factor and request of the resident.

I think they have a party here at night, it is so loud

Many stories about nursing home experiences leave me awestruck. The environment and culture of a facility will vary. Depending on the acoustics in the facility (tiled floor versus carpeted) you may hear every sound. If floors are tiled and uneven, the nurse's medication cart rolling down the hallway can sound like a Mack truck. A carpet cleaning that occurs at night when most residents are sleeping and not walking around can be deafening.

A carpet cleaning can certainly occur during the day instead of late at night. If the noise is a matter of rambunctious staff, the management should be informed and can address the issue through staff education and accountability.

I do not have any privacy

A private room inherently affords a person more privacy than a semi-private or group room arrangement. Did you know that during state health surveys the inspectors monitor if staff knocks on patient doors __and__ wait for an acknowledgement from the patient before entering? The consistent use of this practice is a matter of facility expectations and staff accountability. Further, if you find staff consistently leaving doors open during personal care sessions or staff not knocking on the door, request a meeting with the administrator and nursing management to discuss these issues and request they add your preferences to your care plan.   You can also express these concerns during the resident council and family meeting that your activities director facilities.   The Resident and Family Council meetings are an opportunity to discuss (in a group) the improvements the facility needs to consider.

The wheelchair is always dirty

A common practice, though inconsistent, is for the washing of wheelchairs while patients are resting.   Washing a wheelchair is not a complicated task.   If you notice wheelchairs are dirty with accumulated food or body odors, you might request the facility enforce the wheelchair washing schedule.   You might want to inquire about an established wheelchair-washing schedule.   To confirm consistent exercise of the policy look at the wheelchairs of residents when you tour and visit.   Dirty or smelly chairs imply a non-existent policy or inconsistent observation of that policy.

Your family may never experience anything on this list of common complaints, but if you do, I would encourage you to talk with the management at the facility (administrator and director of nursing) to come to an acceptable resolution.   In the case of inadequate notice, you should follow-up with the Long-term Care Ombudsman program if you feel the facility has not provided adequate notice to the proper person. You can also contest the premise of a discharge.   The long-term care ombudsman can address complaints about a facility's lack of response to your needs or alleged violations of your patient's rights.   If you feel your safety, well-being, and care needs are in jeopardy by all means file an official complaint with the state and without delay move to your secondary facility of choice.

The Coaching Session

How do you feel about the discussion of nursing homes?   Do you feel more comfortable with the facility you plan to use?   Do you and your family have homework to do?   I hope what you feel right now is a mixture of the two.   I want you to feel empowered and comfortable in the knowledge that you can have a direct affect on the quality of your nursing home experience. The way to exert this power is to take control and connect with good nursing home providers before your family is in a crisis.

If you do not currently have several ready resources for nursing home care and/or do not feel comfortable walking into a nursing home and evaluating it, I encourage you to give me a call. My clients recovering from fear and planning paralysis can attest to my ability to "make it happen."

I would suggest at least starting the conversation with your family. Tread carefully though. Some older adults are concerned that once their family gets them into a nursing home they may be tempted to leave them there for self-serving reasons. If you still find resistance from your loved one, I would suggest scheduling a confidential caregiver coaching session with me. Sometimes caregivers benefit from an objective third party hearing their message. As an experienced nursing home professional and elder care specialist I understand your dilemma. I am skilled at facilitating tough conversations with clients, some of them obstinate, and can help you tailor your message and do so in a way that increases receptivity and minimizes your stress. Every caregiver can use less stress and healthier relationships.

Seven

Home Health Care

In Chapter Four I explained the continuum of care and the two types of home health care, medical home health care and private duty (non-medical) home health care. Medical home health care occurs in a traditional home, an independent living apartment or assisted living community, and is therefore available to you almost anywhere you call home (except nursing homes).

Medical home health care is a "skilled" service that requires the expertise of health and medical professionals (i.e. nurse, physical therapist, occupational therapist, speech therapist, social worker, and home health aide). Medicare will pay for all of those skilled professionals to come to your home. Remember the importance of medical necessity for Medicare to reimburse for a health care service. Medical home health care is no exception. In order to receive your Medicare home health care benefits, the following basic qualifiers must be met:

1). A doctor must write an order for you to receive medical home health care.

2). Your medical situation must be such that you require "skilled" services for Medicare to reimburse for medical home health care.

3). You must be "home bound" to continue to see the medical home health care providers. Homebound means you are unable to leave your home or you leave your home primarily for medical appointments, and it is taxing for you to leave your home.

Finding an agency you prefer

How do you go about finding an agency you prefer? The short answer is interview as many agencies as you need until you have at least two agencies with which you are comfortable. You may be thinking to yourself, "Does the hospital do this for me?" Well, yes and no. Hospitals refer to home health agencies they know.

A home health agency tells a hospital what services it provides and the hospital refers patients who need those services. Some home health agencies respond to referrals faster than others do and that is a good thing in a hospital's view. Remember hospitals have many patients to discharge and many new patients who replace those who are discharged. The faster an agency can respond the better.

The hospital cannot assure the quality a home health agency will provide. That responsibility falls to patients and their families. This brings us back to the procedure of how to find a quality home health agency. Word of mouth testimonials from trusted friends, co-workers, and family members are a good place to start. No matter the method you use to find the name and phone number of an agency, you want to take your search a step further. Your careful research, interviews, and critical assessment will help eliminate agencies that do not meet your preferences.

Tools to help make first contact

If you are among the few people who already have the name and number of a couple of preferred home care agencies, good for you. If you do not have an agency in mind that you have researched and trust, keep reading. If you are seeking a medical home health provider that accepts your Medicare insurance, an important tool to use is *Home Health Compare*. Home Health Compare is an online search and home health care comparison tool operated by the federal government. The online tool provides information about the performance of Medicare-certified home health agencies and provides consumers with information about how well, on paper, home health providers are caring for the Medicare patients they serve. By using Home Health Compare, one can find agencies with the precision of a city or zip code. The tool does not profile agencies that are not Medicare certified.

Exceptions are recently certified home health agencies, agencies that strictly accept private insurance, or agencies that do not accept any private or government sponsored insurance at all.

> **CARE TIP**: Many hospitals and medical centers also offer medical home health care and accept Medicare for payment.

To find non-Medicare home health care agencies you can contact elder care locator at www.eldercare.gov or call them toll-free at (800) 677-1116 weekdays, 9:00 a.m. to 8:00 p.m. EST. You can also get local information from your phone book. Keep in mind, neither of these sources provides guidance on making a decision.

What questions should you ask?

As an aside, let me warn that many families assume that the mere fact that an agency or facility is still operating implies that they have had no "serious" problems. This assumption can be far from accurate. I believe the majority of agencies do their best to provide quality care, seek to employ professional and ethical workers, and overall plan to do well at managing patient care. However, many agencies fall short in one area or another.

What should you look for in the interest of connecting with home health providers whose practice reflects the characteristics mentioned above? Let's assume that before you get to this step you have already taken the steps of talking with family, friends, doctors, your hospital, and an elder care specialist about home health agencies. After talking with your trusted confidantes, the agencies on your list should include ones you have a good feeling for, based on the feedback provided by confidants, and on your list should be other agencies you would like to explore but about which you have limited or no history These agencies may be those that you saw or heard in an advertisement.

The first priority is to make sure the agency accepts the insurance you will use to pay for the care. As I said, some agencies accept almost any insurance, others accept Medicare, Medicaid, and still others require a family to pay out-of-pocket for the care and do not accept insurance at all. Once you establish the insurance factor, the next questions relate to detail.

Minimum Acceptable Criteria
Some essential factors that are not negotiable include:

1) The agency offers the services you need. Speech and Occupational Therapists are hard to find in a home health environment. If you need one or both of these professionals you want to make sure the agency employs them or has an established contract with a staffing agency that will provide the therapy staff.

Some companies report they provide all three therapies (occupational, physical and speech), but in reality they provide them by contract and when there is an urgency for therapy the contracts are ineffective and the patients do not get the services they need.

Before you leave the hospital talk with your therapists and doctors about what home health services you should have. Ask your doctor to write a prescription for the recommended services and request that the hospital therapists document the reason for the prescription and describe in general, what they want the home health therapists to evaluate. Make sure you get at least an evaluation from the home health care professionals that the doctors and hospital therapists say you should see. If your doctors and hospital therapists recommend at least an evaluation (one visit) by a specific type of therapist, you should receive the recommended service.

2) The home health agency (or their staffing agency) completes a thorough background check on all of their employees *before* they are assigned to a patient. Some agencies hire staff/employees to provide care. Some agencies use contracts from outside agencies to provide workers. Be certain to understand whether the worker is a hired employee or a contracted employee. A manager should have sufficient procedural knowledge to clarify the worker screening process.

There is no inherent problem with using a staffing agency. You do want to understand the employee background check and screening process undertaken for the professionals who come into your home. Further, ask specifics about the background check procedures. Inquire as to whether the background check includes violations from within the state where you reside or if employees undergo a national background check (FBI background check) which will search for offenses completed anywhere in the entire U.S.

Some predators move from state to state and therefore remain undetected. This background check information is necessary to have for the nursing home and home health settings. I share this information with you not to raise alarms, the reality is that seniors in particular are vulnerable and predators are aware of that vulnerability. Reputable and responsible agencies should provide for state and national background checks.

3) The employees wear name badges and use proper protective equipment when working with your loved one (i.e. wears gloves and washes hands before and after treatments). All agencies are required to have a standard operating procedure in this area. After many years in health care, I am amazed by the unsanitary behavior I have observed from seemingly smart professionals. I will spare you the worst of the details, but let me say, you want to make sure people wash their hands upon entering your home, and certainly before touching your wounds or providing direct care to you or a loved one.

I remember my own health care experience where I was challenged to practice what I preach. A few years ago, I had to seek medical treatment. The kind and friendly nurse entered the room and quickly donned gloves, without washing her hands. That was the first significant part of it. She was professional and engaging as she talked with me and proceeded to walk around to the right side of my bed. All the while, she was dragging her gloved right hand along the bedrail then she reached to open the IV package. I could not believe it. Before she touched the packaging, I said, as softly as I could manage, "Can you please change your gloves?" To which she replied, "These are clean, I just put them on." To myself, I thought, "maybe they were before you dragged them along the ER hospital bed rail" and God only knows what body fluids had been on that thing! Instead, I calmly explained why I wanted her to change the gloves, and she had no idea what her hands were doing at the time and apologized profusely. Some of you might be saying to yourselves that I am being fussy because, after all, they wash down the ER beds. It is the practice that rooms and beds *should* be cleaned, and maybe they are.   Nevertheless, I was not taking any chances.

You cannot protect yourself from all germs, but some very dangerous diseases are transmitted in the health care settings due to lack of hand washing, improper glove use, and other sanitization and sterilization issues. Do not ever hesitate to speak up for yourself and your health. By the way, you should never have to apologize for doing so.

4) Ask about staffing levels to evaluate if the agency has adequate staff to provide a requested service within a matter of a few days, not weeks. If you need a nurse and the company only has one nurse servicing the entire geographic area this could be problematic during a scheduling crunch and may mean some missed visits for you.

5) Make sure the agency covers your geographic area frequently and that inconvenient travel does not preclude your getting the care you need. This is especially important for those living in rural areas. As a home health occupational therapist, I remember traveling over 60 miles *one-way* to see a patient for an agency because nobody else would go. Fortunately, the person did not need regular occupational therapy services, and two visits were sufficient. If you live in a rural area and have difficulty getting services make sure you understand ahead of time how the excess travel may affect the frequency you are seen. While where you live should not affect the frequency of your care, in reality, it could and you should ask about it beforehand.

When you are going through the interview process, enter the conversation with written questions and document the responses so you can refer to them later. If you commit to interviewing several agencies, it will be helpful to keep things organized and separate by documenting each interview in writing. Questions you ask should relate specifically to the care you want and, if appropriate, the medical care you need.

Beyond the Basics

If during the interview, the agency receives passing marks on the basics, you can proceed to the questions that help you predict quality of care. Obviously, if the agency fails on the basics, you can consider the conversation closed, unless of course you just want to practice your interview skills.

So what are some questions to ask to help you predict the type and quality of care you may receive with each of the agencies you are interviewing? These questions are the fundamentals of an interview. An agency may be good for a medical need related to a pressure wound and not so good for a medical need related to a hand injury.

The basis for all of the quality questions relates to your medical or situational needs.

Components of the qualitative assessment include:

1) Asking about the skill level and expertise of the person providing the care. For example, most nurses are familiar with how to dress and treat a wound and can certainly follow a physician's order on applying a wound cover.

The difference in terms of care is, for example, a nurse who can perform the technical aspects of wound care well versus a *nurse wound care specialist*. A nurse wound care specialist, because of special training, classes, experience or certifications, can provide alternative treatment suggestions and bring to bear more progressive treatment options that may work better, faster, or more effectively. You, as a patient, may never know the difference unless you ask about the training and experience and consider it when evaluating the agencies and professionals who work for them.

2) Ask how field staff communicates with each other about your care? I cannot underscore enough the importance of communication between medical and health care staff. A clinician's job is easier and more effective if performed on a team of professionals who have different experience and expertise. Team members communicate progress, collaborate to solve challenges, and communicate changes in their schedules and appointments that a patient may have set.

By asking about procedural communication methods, you want to know how and with what frequency the professionals communicate with each other about your care since the communication and solidarity of the team can affect the quality of care you receive.

3) Ask how the agency compares with and ranks among the top agencies in your area. Health care providers who are concerned about their performance typically attempt to perform better. Agencies should have quality improvement departments or dedicated staff whose task is to guide the agency in working smarter, more efficiently, and more productively from a business perspective. This department should also help the agency identify areas of improvement related to patient care.

For example, a quality improvement focus may be decreasing the number of patients who go to the hospital ER, decreasing the number of patients with high pain levels, or increasing the number of patients who are able to get to and from the shower independently. All of these areas, in part, demonstrate the effectiveness of the home health care treatments and visits.

An agency that is committed to quality improvement and better patient care will have structures and procedures in place to continually monitor problems and develop effective solutions. The methods for each agency varies based on budget and, frankly, the priority they place on improving performance and assuring quality. Agencies can outsource all or part of the quality improvement process and can elect to routinely get detailed comparison reports and consumer surveys about their performance.

Other methods include having internal departments that manage one component of quality improvement and delegating some parts of the process to outside consulting firms. The method of evaluating improvement and quality can affect the validity of the data, but you want to know that the agency has a demonstrated value for quality improvement, is looking at it, and is effective in implementing solutions and improving quality.

4). If, for whatever reason, an appointment is missed what is the agency's established procedure and actual record for making up missed visits? Schedules are an outline for the things we plan to accomplish. In reality, patients, therapists, and nurses get sick, have sick children, face inclement weather, or forget to communicate a doctor's appointment. All of these scenarios can contribute to a patient not receiving a scheduled visit.

Because home care workers travel, sometimes throughout a large geographic area, rescheduling a visit can be more complicated than it sounds. At the very least, you want to have someone from the agency see you in the interim. If your primary health care worker cannot see you, learn the available options of having a substitute home care worker see you so that you get the frequency of treatments that were initially recommended.

The basic and quality assessment areas I mentioned should provide you with a good amount of information about an agency's staffing patterns, help identify its operating procedures, help you assess the value an agency places on quality and improving performance, and inform you about an agency's specific ability to care for your individual needs. If you complete the planning process before you accept or seek home health care services, you and your family should be quite familiar and comfortable with the agency you choose.

Comparing the Competition

A popular auto insurance company runs commercials that tout their company will help you compare auto insurance premiums. Essentially, they will provide you with sample quotes from their competitors in the auto insurance industry to see if their auto insurance will be the better choice for you. While I do not know how the company produces the numbers from the competitors, the concept seems to have appeal. Why not ask a potential medical home health care provider how they compare in the issues that matter most to you?

Medical home health care agencies have access to reports that tell them exactly where they rank among the agencies in your area on their ability to improve wounds and increase a patient's skills in bathing, toileting, and other activities of daily living. These numbers are typically derived from health data that agencies complete. Sometimes the companies you least expect are on the bottom in key categories. Sometimes a low rating is related to staff choosing the wrong box on a checklist, other times a low score is warranted because a patient has not improved significantly in a key area of care (such as wounds, walking, pain level, bathing, or other areas of self care).

If you ask an agency for details about its ranking and a representative reports that information is privileged, ask what they *can* tell you about their outcomes and effectiveness. You may get a superlative answer like "We are very good," which means little to nothing. Alternatively, you may get a true response about the programs they have in place to address issues with wounds or the training of the staff about hip replacement protocols, for example.

I would not anticipate receiving unflattering reports from the agency itself, but the answers and the way in which your question is addressed may enlighten you as to the agency's philosophy on quality of care and style in managing consumer concerns and complaints. Actively seek to get all the information you can to make a well-informed decision. As you know, getting there is part of the effort; staying there is another part.

Managing the Experience

Here are a few quick tips to make your home health experience more productive and easier on your household.

1). When your doctor decides medical home health care is appropriate, get the phone number for the agency in writing. If you completed the planning process that I just described, you will be the one telling the hospital which provider you prefer and you can share the contact information with them. What a welcome change of pace!

2). Call the agency office and get the name of the person who writes the schedule and assigns visits. This person will be a good contact when you need to know if a home health care worker is planning a trip to your home.

3). Identify which home care worker is assigned (i.e., nurse or physical therapist), and the expected day and time of your first visit. This can help you decide if you need extra supplies in the interim. If the nurse plans to come out to your home the same day you are released from the hospital, you may get the supplies you need for a wound or machine from him or her.

4). Always keep a calendar readily available for home care workers to write their next appointment. During my years as a home health care therapist, I have seen many families get frustrated with the multiple visits involved with home health care. Realize the bombardment is temporary. Your life and household will return to normal very soon. In the meantime, make it easier to adapt your personal appointments and business/work appointments to the home health care schedule by requiring that home health care workers write their next appointment on the calendar and call you in a timely manner if they need to cancel.

5). If your schedule requires home health workers to visit unsupervised, leave a pencil and pad available for notes and reports. Communicate at the onset that you would like to know how things are progressing and how your loved one performed with the areas that have been identified as needing improvement. If the patient is having trouble walking and has to climb stairs, the note taking is a good way to monitor progress and you will have a history of what activities have been focuses for the therapists and/or nurses.

This can help you track what issues have been addressed adequately. Having this information will help you frame intelligent conversations with the agency about the plan of treatment and strategize discharge plans and timeframes. Also the information can potentially strengthen your requests for additional services if you find requesting ongoing care is appropriate.

6). If possible, get the contact information for each home care worker. Some home care workers do not provide their personal cell phone numbers. However, you should be aware of an alternate way to contact them if needed, such as a pager or office number. Having contact information readily available will make it much easier to confirm schedules, change visit times, request supplies, and ask questions if you are not present for a visit.

Balance the Focus on Depth and Breadth (Size)

You may be wondering about advice on size and number of employees. These are important but keep this in mind; health care professionals (nurses and therapists who feel they can do a better job) start some home care agencies. Some agencies you encounter will be new and some agencies offer boutique (highly specialized) services. Look at the overall quality of the agency rather than the size or length of time in business.

Regardless of the length of time in business or the size of the agency, the criteria for what you perceive as quality and the methods you use to find it should be the same. At the end of the evaluation process, a smaller or boutique agency may prove to work best for you.

Location, Location, Location

Bigger and prettier does not necessarily mean greater commitment to quality of care. Do not make your decision solely based on façade or presentation. Think about businesses you know with prime real estate, yet would not recommend them nor entrust the care of a loved one to their service. As you carry out your commitment to planning for home health care, you will find some unexpected surprises along the way that reflect this idea. Consider yourself fortunate to discover these truths from an academic standpoint during planning rather than once you have committed. Since the home health workers will come to you, the location should not be more important than the quality of care the agency can deliver.

In terms of location, you want to make sure the agency has a secure means of safeguarding your personal information. Securing patient information should be a priority and is a legal requirement for all health care providers. Security of personal and health information is more a matter of procedure than office location.

What if…

You want to hope and plan for the best-case scenario, which often translates to more hope than plan. What if you did not establish a plan; did not follow your instincts during the planning process; or you are misled by a good salesperson? What should you do to end the relationship or manage the worst-case scenario?

If you are paying privately, you can leave at your will, as with private duty home care. If Medicare is paying for the services, first I hope that you talk with the agency management to see if you could *work out the kinks*. If that is not possible, realize that your benefits belong to you and under most circumstances; you can walk-away from one provider and begin a relationship with another as long as you qualify for the health care service you are seeking and the new provider accepts your insurance. This is possible even during the middle of a home care experience.

> **CARE TIP**: If you have insurance other than Medicare or Medicaid, talk with your insurance provider about restrictions related to transferring to another agency.

If, after using your skills at diplomacy, transferring your care is the only option on the table, be certain to contact you doctor to inform him or her of your plans before you alert anyone at the current agency of your intent to transfer. Frankly, if you have already shared your concerns with the agency, you should not have to threaten to leave in order to get results.

If you do want to transfer, explain to your doctor the reason(s) you are seeking the transfer and most likely he or she will support your valid reasons or advise you otherwise if you are missing a critical aspect. Your doctor's office contacting the current provider can expedite the current home care agency taking the procedural discharge steps needed to transfer your care to a different agency.

If you feel the care you receive is substandard, exercise your right to go elsewhere. There is no advantage to remaining dissatisfied. The home health agency's unsatisfied customer may never come back and because of your less than ideal experience, you may not refer anyone else. I am sure the agency will be most apologetic and may redeem itself by not causing delays. A word of advice, plan a transfer well so that you will not miss any critical visits (wound care treatments or vital medical interventions).

The Coaching Session

Where nursing care is concerned you may not get the same nurse every time. Your therapy caregiver may be more consistent, though therapist assistants require a supervisory visit from a "therapist" on a routine basis as required by the state. If building a relationship with a nurse or therapist is important inquire about how the home health agency manages assignments. In some agencies you can rotate through 4-5 nurses, at other agencies you are assigned one nurse, and others see you only if your regular caregiver is not available. Know your preferences and express them during your interview of home health agencies. You should know that if one agency is not fulfilling your needs, you can transfer your care to your secondary agency of choice, as appropriate.

Eight

Documenting Your Wishes

Let's assume you are motivated and follow-through on the planning guidance provided here. You screen providers for each level of care and connect with resources to provide the support you need to Age in Place (at home). You may even realize the benefit of seeking professional support. All of those strategies are very important to ensure a quality long-term living experience, but what about the issues over which you cannot actively exert control? Life is a dynamic experience, for which we should do our best to develop contingency plans, but essentially we do not control the journey.

The list of circumstances over which we have no control is fairly long. We all expect to be able to express our concerns and advocate for our best interests but what happens when a health related life event robs us of the ability to self advocate? Tools that you need to address unpredictable life events are the legal documents that express preferences when you cannot. The documents do not have to be expensive to prepare. As a matter of fact, some states offer free forms on their state website. In most states, there are legal aide services for the poor. Depending on the intricacies of a situation, an attorney in a general law practice can draft many of the standard documents for a minimal fee.

Issues that keep families from planning in a timely fashion include:
1) Cost. You know that attorney's fees are not necessarily "cheap." Attorneys have knowledge and an expertise of the law that most people simply do not. Consumers who cannot imagine reading and understanding the law pay attorneys for their knowledge, education,

and skill. Like them or not, good attorneys are worth more than your standard purchase. With that in mind, the question to ask yourself is "how much it is worth to protect my family and my health care wishes?"

In reality, legal, financial, and elder care specialists offer families a value that outweighs the cost of their services. When evaluating the cost of legal documents and elder care consulting, the equation should be a matter of cost-benefit and added value, not merely a function of dollar amounts.

2) Time. You are busy and believe you cannot possibly find the time to get additional things done. While I would prefer you get it all done, try setting a timeline and commit to doing a couple of things at a time. If needed, spread the process out over the course of a couple of weeks or months. The goal is to get the documents in place sooner rather than later.

3) The assumption that everyone already knows your preferences. As I will detail later in this chapter, verbal communication is an important part of making sure your health care wishes are observed, but the hospital cannot take action based on what someone else says you said. When talking about potentially life altering and life ending decisions, *he said she said* may not satisfy a physician and, potentially, not the courts if it progresses to that level.

Much like insurance, you cannot calculate the value of having legal documents in place until you actually need them. How thankful are you when after an automobile accident you can produce a valid insurance card to cover any damages for which you may be responsible or simply to provide proof of insurance to the responding police officer and avoid a ticket? I am not exercising a flair for the dramatic. The reality is that dramatic and catastrophic events can rob anyone of their ability to speak for themselves. In this case, truth is much more dramatic than anything we can imagine, especially when it is real for us.

The essential documents your family needs to have in order to ensure your estate, health care, and legal wishes are carried out even if you cannot speak for yourself include, at a minimum, a will and advanced directives.

Advanced Directives

While a will is the document that after death instructs survivors and heirs what to do with one's belongings, an advanced directive provides guidelines for decisions made in life. Advanced directives are legally enforceable directions that you provide in advance of being in a health care situation where you are unable to speak for yourself. In this situation, the advance directive communicates your wishes for you.

Types of advanced directives are: living will, health care proxy, and power of attorney documents. Each state determines what components should be included in the advanced directive documents.

Health care institutions are now required by law to inquire if you currently have an advanced directive and if you would like to initiate one. In defining the three main types of advanced directives, I'm sure you will see the benefit each has to you and your interests.

If this, then that...

A living will is a written legal document that specifies which types of medical interventions you desire should you not be able to speak for yourself. For example, a living will might state, "If a physician determines my condition, disease, or illness is incurable and terminal, I do not want life-sustaining measures if the sole purpose of those measures is to prevent death."

The living will can be as specific as to certain treatments, or the more common element is the provision for the use of life- sustaining measures, including the use of Cardiopulmonary Resuscitation (CPR) or the use of artificial respiration, and mechanical feeding. A real life example of this is a case in which the brain does not control even involuntary body functions, but machines and artificial ventilation can keep one technically alive though unresponsive and unlikely to recover. A living will directs medical professionals if these measures should be initiated and/or discontinued.

Recently there have been highly publicized cases about verbally communicated health care preferences. Perhaps you have been motivated by those cases to talk with your loved one about your preferences. Most of you have pre-determined if you want to live long-term by artificial means and you should communicate those preferences to the people who may need to talk with your medical professionals on your behalf. While it is important to clearly communicate preferences to family members and potential surrogate decision makers, it is equally important to document those wishes.

If you do not document your wishes you run the risk of having your loved ones not agree among on a course of action or you run the risk of a single decision maker not following through on what you thought you clearly communicated. If you have siblings you can certainly understand how getting people to agree on a course of action for parents may be difficult if not nearly impossible. The issue becomes what the doctors and medical professionals should do if there is disagreement among the parties.

If you have a living will, generally, the preferences outlined in the living will take precedence. If you do not have a living will, the hospital may legally have to take action that reflects your children's decision, even if that decision differs from what you verbally communicated to your children, but neglected to document for the reference of health care professionals.

If you or your loved one have a conviction about mechanical means of life support or other medical interventions, I highly encourage you to establish a living will. It is a dynamic document that you as the person establishing the will can modify. The best way to ensure your wishes are fulfilled, even if you cannot speak for yourself, is to allow your pre-established documents to speak for you.

Who Manages Your Business

A power of attorney is a legal written document that allows you to appoint a surrogate decision maker in the event that you are medically unable to make decisions for yourself. A power of attorney will have the ability to make decisions on legal transactions, sales and purchases, and general business on your behalf, such as cashing checks and paying bills.

I have seen power of attorney documents where one person handled day-to-day money management and another person made decisions about investments. The lawyer drafting the power of attorney can structure it with multiple people being power of attorney and require them to agree before a decision is made, or have one person managing everything, or several people who have different roles and function independently within those roles (i.e., finance and health care).

The power of attorney document is not about giving control to someone else, it is a way to ensure your preferences are executed and financial business is conducted even if you cannot speak for yourself. The choice of who you assign as power of attorney is an important one. The person you choose to manage your finances can have broad control over your money. For this reason, it is advisable to choose a trusted friend or family member. You can revoke the power of attorney at any time, unless you are legally and medically determined incompetent.

The major types of Powers of Attorney are:

1). Non-durable – allows for a person to act on your behalf for financial and business decisions for a specific situation or for a specific period of time.

2). Durable – allows a person to act for you even before you become completely incapacitated or incapable of making financial or business decisions on your own.

3). Springing – only takes effect after a certain predetermined event occurs.

Each state has laws determining what should be included in power of attorney documents. If you do not have a power of attorney document, the hospital can draft one for you upon admission, but I would not wait until a hospital admission to establish it. Your need for hospitalization may be such that you are not able to make a sound decision, and as a result, negate your ability to establish a power of attorney on your own terms.

Power of attorney documents are legally binding and must meet certain statutory (legal) requirements. For this reason, it is not advisable to print generic online documents that may not cover the requirements for the state in which you reside. Some states offer general forms online that comply with their state statutes.

State laws governing advanced directives change. A document drafted 10 years ago may not cover all current legal provisions. Estate planning attorneys recommend you have the documents reviewed for current statutory compliance every 5 years or so and as changes in your life dictate. If your advanced directive is more than 5 years old, consider having an attorney review it for compliance.

Who Manages Your Health Care

A health care proxy is a legal document that assigns a surrogate decision maker. This other person will make medical decisions in the event you are unable to make decisions yourself. The health care proxy takes effect due to medical incapacity or mental incompetence. A health care proxy is often referred to as a medical or health care power of attorney.

The person functioning as your health care proxy has the right to make medical decisions for you. This includes choosing, refusing, and discontinuing treatment. This person should have a clear understanding of your medical preferences and the circumstances under which you would make a certain decision (i.e. refusing mechanical feeding or removing life support).

One's next of kin (a spouse, parent, or adult child) can informally function as a surrogate decision maker without a formal health care proxy. However, it is advisable to have formal documents that clearly communicate your preferences. In addition to documenting your preferences, you should talk with your family and surrogate decision makers about those preferences.

In my experience, most surrogate medical decision makers want to make the right decision; the right decision being that which their loved one would prefer. By clearly communicating your preferences in advance, your family and health care professionals will do a better job in serving your interests, should you be unable to direct them.

The best way to ensure decision makers observe your wishes is to document your preferences and verbally communicate those preferences. Both the informal conversation with surrogate decision makers and providing written documentation ensure the execution of your health care preferences. This communication should occur well in advance of needing someone to act on your behalf. People tell you along the way what they prefer. Such informal conversations are often sparked by news stories, movies, and family events. Despite informal communication, the emotional heat of the moment can prevent objective decision making by a loved one. The legal documentation is insurance.

A situation in my personal life illustrates why both the documents and the communication are so important. I frequently talk with my pop about long-term care and aging. He is 70 and has many concerns about age related changes. Part of the concern relates to fear of Alzheimer's and the inability to make independent decisions. Every forgotten word or lost thought is cause for alarm to those who have a mastery of words and characters of fierce independence. My dad is that guy!

During our conversations, he rarely fails to communicate the idea that he does not want to live if unable to make decisions for himself. I don't know that any of us would follow his wishes without temptation to act from an emotional level and second guessing his preferences.

The emotional aspect is difficult, especially if it is an end-of-life decision. Who wouldn't immediately respond with emotion? By documenting your preferences, you are in effect directing your decision makers. As a surrogate decision maker, there is immeasurable peace in knowing you are doing exactly what your loved one prefers.

Two well publicized cases illustrate the importance of advanced directives and estate planning documents. They are the cases of Anna Nicole Smith and Terri Schiavo.

According to her ex-husband, Terri Schiavo informed him of her desire to not have artificial and mechanical life support if the sole purpose was to keep her alive. This preference was reportedly communicated when she was healthy and able to make decisions for herself. The test of this informal communication came after she suffered a heart attack and became dependent on mechanical means of support. Without a documented advanced directive or health care proxy, the case spiraled into a very public court battle. Florida's governor, the Florida State Supreme Court, and US legislature all attempted to force a resolution. In fact, the US Senate and Congress unsuccessfully attempted to force hearing of the case by the US Supreme Court. Mrs. Schiavo's wishes, as communicated by her husband, were eventually honored, after many years of battle. Remember the passionate opposing arguments of her husband and parents? I do not presume to offer an opinion about who was "right" in this family conflict. The reality is; an advanced directive would have clearly communicated Terri's wishes.

While Mrs. Schiavo's case is a demonstration of how adults of all ages, young and old, should consider advanced directives for health care, Anna Nicole Smith's situation reflects that youth is not exempt from needing estate planning documents.   Ms. Smith's estate plan, as reported, also underscores the importance of updating legal documents to reflect current preferences, life circumstances, and family situation. In Anna Nicole's case, her will only covered her son, and explicitly left no provision for any other children or potential heirs.   Unfortunately, her son died shortly after her daughter was born.   Ms. Smith herself expired before she changed her will to provide financially for her new daughter and the millions of dollars her infant daughter could potentially inherit.

In a society that favors youth, one expects longevity.   The reality is, accidents happen and the consequences of risky behavior can be irrevocable.   Everyone, regardless of age, should have advanced directives, a will, and a trust if appropriate.

I must confess: it took some time to institute my own estate plan and health care directives.   Every time I looked at my own family, or informed someone else's family about the importance of legal documents, I felt a twinge of guilt.   I can tell you, knowing that I have made legal provisions for my family is comforting.   Documenting the preferences I have informally communicated to family offers a peace of mind that I encourage you to seek if you have not already.

An advanced directive is a straight forward document. Depending on the complexity of one's estate (the number of heirs, preference in dividing property and belongings, and other personal estate planning instructions) a will can be simple or complex.   A qualified attorney (or the hospital) can guide you in establishing an advanced directive that meets the requirements for your state.   An attorney can help your family devise a comprehensive last will and testament.

I encourage you to make several copies of your advanced directives as every health care provider you work with will request a copy for their records.   Since your advanced directives will inform the types of care that are allowed and will communicate your preference for heroic medical interventions, the health care providers need to have documentation on site.   This onsite documentation will justify actions taken by the provider or the lack of action taken, as the case may be.

Guardianship

Before we close this chapter I what to mention two additional legal tools. They are guardianship and a trust.

A guardianship is awarded by the courts when a person is considered incompetent to make decisions. Guardianship can be awarded to a family member, friend, or to an attorney, if no suitable alternative is available. Guardianship often becomes an issue when a person makes self-destructive decisions that jeopardize his/her health and/or the health and well-being of others. Guardianship requires that the person undergo assessment and be deemed incompetent. Without such proof of incompetence the courts will not forcibly remove one's right to make decisions for him/herself.

A person may contest a request for guardianship by another individual. If the potential ward (the allegedly incompetent person) fights the request for guardianship a hearing will be held to determine if guardianship is appropriate.

Guardianship may be a tool available to a family, if the person one is caring for is demonstrating self-destructive behaviors. Other circumstances include a history of violence, crippling and uncontrolled mental illness, and other issues that impede sound independent decision making.

Seeking guardianship can be hard on family relationships, especially if the potential ward is resistant to the guardianship request. Under this circumstance, a guardianship hearing can be unpleasant, to say the least. Few people would respond well to the accusation of being unfit to make decisions for him/herself, no matter how apparently true that assessment may be.

Living Trusts

A living trust is a legal document assigning your assets (home, investments, and cash) to you or someone else in an established fashion throughout a lifetime. You can name yourself as trustee and actively manage the assets.

In properly planning for the possibility of incapacitation, the trust document should allow for and identify the successor trustee(s) who can make decisions about the trust on your behalf. The trust can be administered by someone you choose or in the case of guardianship, the trustee may be assigned by the court.

Living Trusts can be for a specific amount of time (during an extended hospitalization) or for the remainder of life. A revocable living trust essentially provides another person the ability to temporarily carryout your financial affairs on your behalf. An irrevocable living trust provides that the assets transferred into the trust remain there permanently, and the recipient of the trust may receive income or benefits from the trust throughout his/her lifetime.

Ordinarily, heirs and survivors receive the remainder of the trust upon one's death, unless the trust agreement establishes a perpetual trust. A perpetual trust is theoretically never-ending. The circumstances under which a trust can be dissolved are included within the trust agreement.

Trusts are established for many reasons and serve many purposes. The goal in establishing the trust will inform how and by whom the trust is operated and under what circumstances it may be changed or dissolved.

Trusts are very complex estate planning tools. One should consult several qualified attorneys experienced in trust establishment and management. Since the rules of a trust can be very nuanced, I would ask a couple of attorneys to discover if there is a consensus on a recommended course of action. Where a trust is concerned, establishing the wrong structure can be costly to correct. If you have two opinions and they differ significantly, seek a third or fourth opinion. If you need assistance locating a qualified elder law attorney in your area, I would suggest speaking with the American Bar Association at (800) 285-2221.

Organization and Storage

Has your spouse or parent ever asked you to get paperwork for him that is "supposed" to be located in the top drawer on the right side in the very back under the blue folder? If the road map to your important documents requires such effort, you need a new system. There are several ways to streamline your document filing and storage. The key is to get a real system. It does not have to be an elaborate or expensive system. You can even use the materials you have at home. Here are several suggestions on getting your documents and long-term care planning files organized.

1. A simple manila folder with all relevant papers clipped or stapled with an indicator of what each group of documents is. A trivia fact that will keep your documents looking clean: fluorescent yellow highlighters are invisible during photocopying. Most other colors including primary yellow show marks or the actual word when photocopied.

2. A Binder Storage System. You can purchase binders and planners that are specifically made for caregivers and older adults to manage appointments, budget, and file documents.

3. Scan documents onto a compact disc. Technology has changed the way we live our lives. Everything from buying a hamburger, paying for gas, to paying our taxes is touched and even directed by technology. Tax filing forms are now on a compact disc instead of being folded, stapled, and stored in a paper envelope.

4. A fire proof safe. Obviously, fire and water do not mix well with valuable documents. A fire and waterproof safe will protect your paperwork from both of these dangers.

5. A safe deposit box. Of course it will cost you to rent the box. The security and peace of mind in knowing your valuable documents are protected may be worth it.

Decide which organization option is best for you. The point is to get organized so that your documents are stored securely and can be easily located by you or someone who will make decisions on your behalf.

Securing Your Information

Families need to have documents available when loved ones need access to them, but be certain to safely discard outdated sensitive documents, sensitive junk mail, old bills, and other items with personal indentifying information.

I do not recommend making copies of a social security card, and you should certainly not indiscriminately allow copies to be made by others. Identity theft is a nearly 60 billion dollar per year business in the United States alone.[1] Safeguard your social security card *and* your Medicare card, since the numbers are usually the same. Your social security number is a straight-line into your credit report and the ability for someone to fraudulently open credit cards and finance purchases in your name.

Request that your creditors, health care organizations, and physician's offices truncate your social security number except for essential communications. Truncating the number means only the last four digits are visible. At least that way a criminal will have to work harder to find the entire number and use your identity.

On the same topic of securing your identity information, every home should have a shredder. The Better Business Bureau reports that thirty-six percent of identify theft occurs by someone the victim can identify and the opportunity and ability to access personal information is a factor.[2] I suggest shredding credit card solicitations, and anything with bank account numbers and other account numbers including medical and utility bills. Information with a social security number or birth date should not reach the trash can without first going through a shredder. The same precaution applies to insurance cards and old credit cards which should be cut into pieces so that the account number is not intact. In today's world, a healthy sense of self preservation serves you well.

Nine

A Personal Note

Connecting with timely resources and support is a necessity in managing the responsibility of elder care and aging services. It may *seem* as easy as addressing the needs that you see. An adequate plan is far more comprehensive than that. Sometimes family members are too close to a situation to see things objectively. What about the rest of the story? Believe me, there is more than meets the eye.

The road of health care and aging is bumpy and it is impossible to predict what lies ahead. I encourage you and your family to not only hope for the best but to plan for it as well. In addition to having an ideal for your retirement life, such as aging in place (at home) or having the best quality nursing home experience, take things a step further by contingency planning for the worst case scenario or least desirable situation.

Some of you may have a mix of tools already in place and other tools you have yet to acquire. If you have all of these tools already in place, you are indeed rare. However, if you do not have all the tools in place, the first step is to talk with your loved ones about preferences; theirs and yours. This conversation in itself will cover a lot and hopefully set the stage for a team approach to planning holistically for retirement living. Don't keep to the pattern of silence. If you are having a difficult time getting the conversation started or having a less than productive discourse give me a call and I will help you move forward. I know some of you are *ready to roll* and take decisive action. Good for you. I would caution you to move with precision rather than haste, especially if you are a caregiver to someone else.

Make sure you set timeframes and document a goal (e.g. visit four nursing homes in the next two months) and hold yourself accountable for achieving that goal. Somehow time is moving faster. I don't know how it happened, but days are not as long as they used to be! Before you know it, three months, six months, and then a year has passed and you haven't accomplished what you needed to in adequately preparing your family. If you are fortunate, you won't need the care in the meantime, but what if you do? Set a goal, stick to it, and build an accountability relationship so you can stay focused and on track. Solutions and accountability are my specialty.

During my coaching sessions clients frequently say, "Okay, I have homework to do!" I am glad people get motivated. Realizing the control you actually have over retirement life is empowering. I not only want you to get motivated, I want you to *stay* motivated. The single most effective tool in staying motivated is to *not procrastinate*! Get motivated and then get active by talking with your family and evaluating what you need. I can help you perform a holistic needs assessment.

I often say, "Consumer power is the catalyst for improving the quality of health care." I truly believe that as families get more informed and empowered, the better the care they will accept and as a result the quality of care will improve to meet consumer expectations. If health care consumers know their rights, ask for what they want and realize they can get it, the quality they receive will improve. The fact is informed health care consumers who ask questions, advocate for themselves, and speak up are better satisfied with the outcome of their care decisions.

I cannot over emphasize how important consumer empowerment is in the retirement living process and every age range. You absolutely deserve to live your entire life by design, and I appreciate you giving me the opportunity to guide you in beginning the process. You can do this, and you do not have to do it alone. I am available to help. I can assure you that retirement life planning is a process that is continually underway. Just like life, the unexpected will happen. The difference is now you are prepared and committed to take control where there is an opportunity to do so.

When you hear someone at work or the gym who is confronted with elder care issues (*and you will*) tell him or her to call Pamela at (866) 545-POPE to get control of their elder care situation.

If you have any questions, know that I am available to work with your family, no matter where you live in the United States. You can contact me by phone toll-free at (866) 545-POPE or (314) 830-9000 or by email at lifebydesign@popeinstitute.com. The Pope Institute Senior Care Call Center is available from 8 a.m. to 5 p.m. CST, Monday through Friday.

I welcome a letter or call from you about how *Retirement Life by Design: Living Well with Health, Wisdom and Authenticity* has affected your life. I wish you and your family a wealth of health and a journey that honors your best laid plans. God bless you and all of your efforts.

The Continuum Of Care Simplified

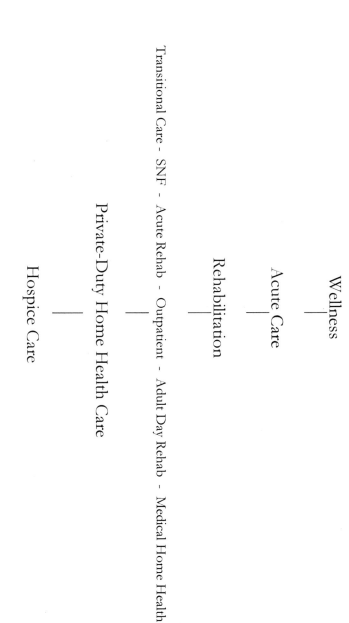

Resources That Can Help

AARP Foundation Grandparent Information Center's (GIC's) Local Grandparent Support Database
AARP (The American Association of Retired Persons) offers a wealth of information for families. Among its least well-know resources is the GIC Local Grandparent Support Database. While AARP does not endorse any of the third party providers in the database, it is a good way to make contact with support groups that may provide respite care, legal assistance, transportation support, and much more. If you are a grandparent functioning as a parent, you can go online to access the support database at http://www.giclocalsupport.org or call AARP directly at (888) 687-2277.

The Alzheimer's Association
Alzheimer's disease is a devastating illness for families and the person diagnosed with it. The mission of the association is a world without Alzheimer's and they provide responsive support to families of a loved one diagnosed with Alzheimer's. Their support services include respite care, education, and family training. To locate a chapter near you visit them online at www.alz.org. If you need support with a loved one with Alzheimer's disease you can contact their 24 hour helpline at (800) 272-3900.

The American Cancer Society
The American Cancer Society offers free lodging (Hope Houses) when cancer survivors need treatment in another state and assistance getting insurance even with a cancer diagnosis. The American Cancer Society helpline is open 24/7 including holidays and is available by calling (800) 227-2345.

The American Parkinson's Disease Association (APDA)

The American Parkinson's Disease Association offers connections to local support groups and meetings, education booklets and materials, transportation support and referrals to physicians who "understand the disease." Some chapters also offer respite care programs. To learn more about the Parkinson's Disease Association and its local programs for your area call (800) 223-2732.

The Amyotrophic Lateral Sclerosis (ALS) Association

The ALS Association has chapters in most major metropolitan areas. The ALS Association offers patient and family education, support services, adaptive equipment, durable medical equipment (DME), and care management services. The services offered at each chapter will vary and are free to those diagnosed with ALS. To locate an ALS chapter near you, go online to www.alsa.org or contact them toll-free at (800) 782-4747.

The Department of Veterans Affairs (VA)

If you are a veteran looking for low-cost health related support, the Veteran's Administration is a good place to start. While there are procedures beneficiaries must follow to access the veteran's support services, the benefits are free and broad in scope. Most veterans I meet have no idea about the broad scope of VA benefits and the steps they need to take to access those benefits.

A sample of benefits available to United State's veterans include: out-patient dental care, home improvement and modifications to make a bathroom accessible, vocational rehabilitation to find and retain gainful employment, burial assistance in government and non-government operated cemeteries, prosthetic and orthotic clinics, wheelchair clinics and much more. You can also call the Veteran's Administration at (800) 827-1000.

Local Heating and Cooling Centers

According to the Centers for Disease Control and Prevention (CDC), between 1979 and 2003, over 8,000 people in the US died from heat exposure. Many older adults, particularly those of lower incomes, and those with poor problem solving are at particular risk of heat exposure.

Many older homes in which seniors reside do not have air conditioning units and even if the home is equipped with air conditioning some seniors avoid running the unit for fear of high utility bills.

I remember advising a nurse who was concerned about her mother who lived with a part-time caregiver but due to confusion would turn off the heating and cooling system regardless of the temperature. The nurse was concerned that her mother could unwittingly expose herself to the elements. The family had purchased a standard thermostat cover which her mom would bypass by using a knife to push and pull the controls. She was confused enough to not weigh the health consequences of changing the thermostat, yet, she was "with it" enough to figure out how to bypass the thermostat cover and change the settings.

To this nurse, I suggested a thermostat cover and digital thermostat that could be programmed for time and temperature adjustments and because of the control arrangement an object could not manipulate the settings. Alternatively, to prevent tampering, one can simply use a digital thermostat with a keypad lock feature.

In a situation where a senior does not have adequate heating and cooling in the home, a heating and cooling center is most appropriate. To locate a heating and cooling center contact your city hall, or local fire or police department. Usually these climate control centers are available during extreme weather (heat waves and power outages during a winter storm). Local churches, health centers, and community centers may function as heating and cooling centers. I would advise residents to check with their local police and/or fire department during severe weather to confirm the location of heating and cooling centers. This may be especially important if you are concerned about a loved one you cannot monitor during such events. Some municipalities may even offer transportation.

Meals on Wheels Association of America

The Meals on Wheels Association offers delivered meals to seniors who continue to live in the community. The meals are delivered in various frequencies and meet nutritional and some disease specific guidelines. The local programs are often administered through churches, health care organizations, and food pantries. To find a Meals on Wheels center go online to www.mowaa.org or call Meals on Wheels at (703) 545-5558.

The National Center on Elder Abuse

The NCEA is a part of the National Administration on Aging. The NCEA works in collaboration with national, state, and local affiliates to prevent and track elder abuse in the US. The Adult Protective Services arm of NCEA responds to and investigates allegations and reports of suspected abuse.

Research suggests only 1 in 14 abuse cases are reported.[1] If you suspect abuse in a home or facility, please contact Adult Protective Services in your area to report the suspected abuse. In filing a report, you are reporting what you suspect is abuse and the investigators will follow-up as appropriate. To file a report of suspected abuse call (800) 677-1116. If you observe a situation that suggests an immediate danger to any one, regardless of age, call 911.

The National Multiple Sclerosis Society (MS)

The MS Society is a major advocate for research, treatment, and cure for people with Multiple Sclerosis. The program and support services offered by the MS Society vary with each chapter. To locate a chapter near you visit the National MS Society online at them toll-free at (800) 344-4867 or go online to www.nationalmssociety.org.

The National Parkinson's Foundation (NPF)

The NPF advocates for research, treatment, education of family caregivers and health care professionals. The NFP offers equipment loan closets for low-to-no cost durable medical equipment, assistance with caregiver respite, and many other programs.   To locate a chapter near you visit NPF online at www.parkinsons.org or call them toll-free at (800) 327-4545.

Pope Institute for Health and Education, LLC (Pope Institute)

Pope Institute provides elder care and aging in place consultations in person and via telephone throughout the United States and Canada. The mission of Pope Institute is to empower elder care consumers by helping seniors age in place at home and get good facility care when needed. The Retirement Living by Design™ Initiative is a company campaign designed to help seniors and aging adults plan for retirement living with an emphasis on quality of life and aging in place.   Visit Pope Institute online at www.popeinstitute.com for seminar information or for resources on talking to seniors about driving, home safety checklists, and how to prepare your home for a hip or knee surgery, among others. The tools are free to download for personal use. You can contact Pope Institute at (866) 545-7673.

The Society for Progressive Supranuclear Palsy (PSP)

PSP is a fatal, progressive, and degenerative brain disease that has no known cure. Most people have never heard of PSP. I spoke with two women within a matter of two weeks at Pope Institute whose spouses were diagnosed with PSP. Neither of them had previously received information about the existence of the Society for PSP or local support resources for families coping with PSP.

If you have PSP or are a caregiver to someone with PSP, please connect with the PSP society. They will be able to help you connect with support groups and other PSP specific resources in your local area. Due to the progressive nature of PSP, life planning is highly recommended. You can contact The Society for PSP at www.psp.org or by calling them toll-free at (800) 457-4777

NOTES

Chapter One

1. Family Caregiver Alliance. Selected Caregiver Statistics. www.fca.org.

2. Genworth Financial. *Yearly Long-term Care Costs Increase 15% Since 2004 to Nearly $75,000 in 2007 According to Annual Study by Genworth Financial.*

Chapter Two

1. Genworth Financial. *Yearly Long-term Care Costs Increase 15% Since 2004 to Nearly $75,000 in 2007 According to Annual Study by Genworth Financial.*

2. Ibid.

3. Ibid.

4. National Alliance for Caregiving and AARP (1997) Family Caregiving in the US: Findings of a National Survey Washington D.C.

5. The Family Caregiver Alliance. Selected Caregiver Statistics 2005

6. Ibid page 7.

7. Family Caregiver Alliance. Selected Caregiver Statistics.

Chapter Three

1. The New York City Department of Mental Health and Hygiene. Depression Social Isolation and the Urban Elderly, 2006.

2. American Foundation for Suicide Prevention. Facts and Figures: National Statistics www.afp.org

3. Stop Suicide, Inc. Suicide Risk Questionnaire. www.stopsuicide.org

4. The Family Caregiver Alliance. Fact Sheet: Selected Caregiver Statistics. www.caregiver.org .

5. Current Population Survey, Annual Social, and Economic Supplement, "Income, Poverty, and Health Insurance Coverage in the United States: 2005" P60-231, issued August 2006 by the U.S. Bureau of the Census.

7. Genworth Financial. *Yearly Long-term Care Costs Increase 15% Since 2004 to Nearly $75,000 in 2007 According to Annual Study by Genworth Financial.*

8. Ibid.

Chapter Four

1. MetLife Mature Market Institute Releases First National Survey of Adult Day Center Costs with Annual Home Health Care Rates. MetLife Press Release September 26, 2007.

Chapter Five

1. CMS Media Affairs, 30 Million Medicare Beneficiaries Now Receiving Prescription Drug Coverage. 2006

2. The Henry J. Kaiser Family Foundation. "Medicare Fact sheet: The Medicare Prescription Drug Benefit". p. 2. June 2007.

3. Kaiser Daily Health Policy Report Medicare Stand-Alone Drug Plan Premiums To Increase 8.7% in 2008 to $40 Per Month [Oct 01, 2007] cited source Appleby, *USA Today*, 10/1. www.kff.org.

4. Ibid p. 1

5. Ibid p. 2

6. National Center of Health Statistics. Therapeutic Drug Use Statistics 2006, table 93.

7. MetLife Mature Market Institute. The MetLife Market Survey of Nursing Home and Assisted Living Costs. October 2007

8. Ibid.

9. Congressional Budget Office. Financing Long-term Care for the Elderly (2004).

Chapter Six

1. Center for Disease Control and Prevention. Injury Center online. Cited source the National Center for Health Spastics 2006 data.

2. Congressional Budget Office Financing Long-term Care for the Elderly. 2004

3. The New York Times. "At Many Homes, More Profit and Less Nursing" September 23, 2007.

4. Ibid

Chapter Eight

1. Better Business Bureau. The 2006 Identity Fraud Survey Report.

2. Ibid

Chapter Nine

1. National Center on Elder Abuse. Fact Sheet. Elder Abuse Prevalence and Incidence. 2005

About the Author

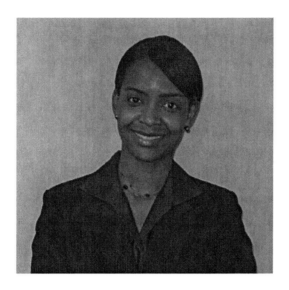

Elder Care and Aging in Place Specialist Pamela Pope uses her experience as a rehabilitation therapist and elder care professional to empower families to manage the challenges of elder care and aging. Her unwavering message of empowerment and holistic planning enlivens her writings and presentations. Pamela Pope brings elder care expertise and an informed advocacy voice to seminars, lectures, and panels on elder care.

As an elder care and aging speaker, Pamela Pope's main topics include

* Aging in Place
* Holistic Retirement Planning
* Innovation and Elder Care Reform

Contact Pamela Pope for speaker requests or interviews at (866) 545-7673 or email ppope@popeinstitute.com. Visit www.popeinstitute.com.

Pope Institute helps families manage elder care challenges with a focus on quality of life and quality of care by providing elder care and aging in place consultations live in selected locations and by phone throughout the U.S. Call (866) 545-POPE to get control of elder care challenges.